STOP KILLING
YOURSELF

STOP KILLING YOURSELF

Make Stress Work for You

Susan Seliger

G. P. PUTNAM'S SONS

NEW YORK

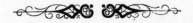

To my mother and father,
To Peter and to Alexander,
May we all live in health

The text of this book is set in 10 pt Times Roman

Library of Congress Cataloging in Publication Data

Seliger, Susan.
Stop killing yourself.

Includes index.
1. Health.   2. Stress (Psychology)—Prevention.
I. Title.
RA776.S454   1984   613   83-24568
ISBN 0-399-12925-1

Illustrations by Barbara McGrath
Book design by Bernard Schleifer

Printed in the United States of America

Acknowledgments

No point in beating about the bush; may as well get to the bottom of things. This book began over a decade ago in London. If Robert Troop and Sylvester Stein hadn't made me editor of their little magazine, *Survival Kit,* that drizzly winter on Upper James Street, who knows what reputable occupation I might have pursued? Instead, I've been a writer on health issues ever since, and I've never looked back—except in gratitude.

Although I have been researching the material in this book for over a decade, the unifying idea did not crystallize until 1978 as I was doing an article for Jack Limpert at *Washingtonian* magazine—and the title comes from Jack as well. The enthusiastic response to that article led me to believe that people were ready to hear a great deal more on the subject.

And my editor at Putnam's, Faith Sale, convinced me further that people would want to hear the information in my voice, not in the voices of the thousands of experts I consulted. It meant that I have left out quotes and the names of the many researchers who generously devoted their time and energy, on the phone and in personal interviews, to discussing their research studies; I am grateful to them all. But more important, Faith's urgings forced me to include only that information that I judged to be the best and most helpful as it would bear the imprint of my voice and I could not hide behind the quote of another. In short, she guided me on the voyage from writing articles to a book; and she did it gently.

For tolerating all the six-day weeks it took to finish this book— Peter, for cheerfully guiding Alexander out of my study, and Alexander, for pleading with Mommy not to go back into that study but to come out and play only half as many times as I know you wanted to say it—to both of you, my thanks are almost as deep as my love.

Of course, if my parents had not instilled in me the desire to "do good" there would be no book.

Finally, I want to thank my grandmother, Essie, may she rest in peace, for repeating so often at the end of her life a phrase that echoed in my head as I wrote: "Listen, as long as you're healthy . . ." She was right; everything depends on that.

Contents

The Big Risks—Fighting the Leading Killers and Cripplers

Introduction

THIS BOOK IS for everyone who would like to get hold of just a little more healthy energy each day.

There is a way.

It is within our power to convert the major energy force in our lives to positive uses. Living, even breathing, everything we do demands constant change, and change evokes a response within us—that response is stress. But it doesn't have to be harmful. Stress is the energy of life. Sometimes it seems to work against us, but we don't have to knuckle under. We can harness that energy force and make it work for us.

When we lose control of that energy, then stress does its dirty work. The systems in our body go haywire: most important, the immune system weakens and leaves us vulnerable to every disease from arthritis to cancer and heart disease, with other unpleasant stops in between. This book explains how you can keep that from happening.

Stress, as most people think of it, is not really the problem. The common thread in the onset of the major killers and cripplers today is not some "stressful" event or even some infectious bug *out there* attacking us. The common thread is *in us*—how we respond to the events of life. The way we behave in each day—what we eat, smoke or drink, how we sleep and exercise, whether we get angry often or laugh instead—can mean the difference between bad stress and good, between getting sick and getting well.

And we have a great deal of control over our responses and, thus, over whether our bodies will dwindle or flow with vital energy.

This is a one-stop health book. I have sifted through thousands of scientific studies and books, spoken to hundreds upon hundreds of experts to distill the information here, not just about how the mind and body work together as an energetic team but also about which tactics have proven most successful in helping people modify their behavior. The book covers both immediate and long-term plans to reduce your health risks and maximize your chances for a happy, healthy life.

Short tests tell you instantly where you stand: whether you are vulnerable to stress, whether your habits are making you old for your age, whether you are at risk for heart disease, or whether you are a Type B or Type A personality who could be headed for heart trouble.

Simple explanations of how the body works and how disease begins equip you to make intelligent decisions on your own about your life and your risks, when you need a doctor and when you can be your own best doctor.

And step-by-step action plans lay out the specific kinds of changes you can make that will bring about the most improvement in your health with the least effort. The Ten-Second Stress Fix, for example, is a technique you can learn to apply in the heat of a stressful experience which enables you to get control of that burst of energy instead of frittering it away nervously. And the illustrated guide to exercises you can do discreetly, without extra effort—in public or in private—can help renew your spirits and your energy and make every spare move count, even for those who hate the whole idea of exercise.

You cannot avoid stress—it is part of life. But you can learn how to convert the bad stress to good. Harnessing your energy for health is the first step you must take if you want to STOP KILLING YOURSELF.

Who's in Charge Here? We Are the Heroes

THE KEY TO GOOD HEALTH lies in understanding how powerfully the mind can influence the body and how easily we can harness that power to fight against illness. We are the heroes in this health saga—not "magic bullet" drugs, machines, or medicine men. And our plan of action for survival against the major killers today must be to prevent them—using mind and body—before they start.

1
The Doctor Within

It's supposed to be a professional secret, but I'll tell you anyway. We doctors do nothing. We only help and encourage the doctor within.
—ALBERT SCHWEITZER

WE FACE A NEW AGE in medical history. We have come to the point where we must reshape our notions of what causes disease and what cures it. It is an age when we ourselves—not doctors or drugs—will come to play the central role in becoming healthy and staying that way.

For the last hundred years since the discovery of microscopic bacteria and viruses, disease was easy to understand. It was a state caused by some mysterious bug that was out there waiting to attack. To get healthy, all one had to do was take a tablet or a shot of one of the latest "magic bullets"—vaccines and antibiotics—that would attack those bugs.

These notions used to make sense. One hundred years ago, a plague could threaten entire cities; and as recently as 1950, the mere rumor of a polio case would throw whole neighborhoods into panic. Vaccines and antibiotics—many discovered only after the 1940s—have virtually eradicated polio, diphtheria, smallpox, tetanus, typhoid, and even measles.

Yet, even with these great strides, many of us are still dying long before our allotted threescore years and ten. For all the wonder drugs and surgical wizardry, a 45-year-old American male today can expect to live only twenty-eight months longer than his counterpart did in 1920. And for many those extra months will not be spent in vigorous activity but in the suffering we've come to expect of old age.

The reason is simple: we're clinging to the false belief that no matter what we do to ourselves—no matter how we eat or drink or push our bodies beyond the limit—if we get really sick, some medical genius somewhere will be able to repair the damage.

But no outside force can fix what's ailing us now.

Most disease that strikes before age seventy is induced by the way we behave. The major killers and cripplers of our time—heart disease, cancer, stroke, diabetes, arthritis, accidents—result not from bugs but from the cumulative effects of our habits and our attitudes as we face the routine stresses of living. It is only through modifying these habits that we will be able to achieve and maintain good health.

It's easy, for example, to say that your boss drives your blood pressure up or that cigarettes cause lung cancer. But the medical truth is far simpler—and harder to accept. The boss, obnoxious though he may be, does not send the blood coursing through your arteries at speeds dangerous enough to lead to a heart attack or stroke, but your *reaction* to him can. Cigarettes lead to the cancerous mutation of lung cells only if you *choose* to smoke them.

The common thread—the cause—is the choices we make. And the cures, for the same reason, lie within ourselves as well. Such simple good habits as having breakfast every day, exercising two to three times a week, getting a decent night's sleep, not smoking, maintaining a moderate weight, have been shown (in a University of California study of over 7000 men and women) to add as much as eleven years to a man's life, seven years to a woman's.

Unfortunately for most of us, changing bad habits isn't easy. Nobody likes to do it. Many of us valiantly try—diets or exercise regimens—only to have to try and try again.

The important thing to bear in mind is that change, like life itself, is not a test that we either pass or fail. Getting 40 percent wrong on a test may have meant F in high school, but in life it means that you've actually gotten 60 percent right. Your body notices and appreciates even tiny improvements—a walk up the stairs instead of an elevator ride, a few cigarettes not smoked, two minutes of stress-reducing deep breathing in the middle of the day. And besides, if one were to gamble on that test score, 60 to 40 odds are better than the best doctor could give you today on surviving, let alone feeling good, once you contract many of the top-ten diseases of our day.

The issue here is not so much staving off death as making our years alive more pleasurable. We are currently a nation of walking wounded: half the thirty-year-old women suffer one or more chronic conditions; 45 percent of men do, too. By the age of sixty, about 60 percent of Americans are stricken by some ailment that brings aches and pains and limits daily activities.

Aging does not have to be this way. We do not have to live in fear of disability in old age. We cannot stop the flow of time but we unquestionably can slow down the deterioration that we have come to expect with its passage.

If we could make only one change in our lives, the most significant would be a change of attitude. It would involve realizing that we, as individuals, actually know ourselves, our mind and body functions, better than any outside expert ever can. Or at least we have that potential. We get minute-by-minute reports of how we're doing. And if we would only pay a little more attention to the signals our body sends out (early-warning signs that will be covered in upcoming chapters), we would know better than any medical specialist when things aren't quite right long before they go seriously awry.

And we *can* do something about it. We should not be intimidated by the medical mystique that only an expert can understand the complexities of the human body and brain. The truth is that no one yet understands those complexities in full. But just because we don't know how things work, or how to cure them when they stop working, doesn't mean we don't know how to prevent them from going out of kilter. The British Royal Navy of the eighteenth century knew nothing about vitamin C and even less about the biochemical mechanisms triggering scurvy, but it recognized that sailors could prevent this deathly disease simply by sucking on enough lemons and oranges.

The medical knowledge is available today—at this very moment without adding a single new discovery—to prevent anywhere from 35 to 75 percent of all cancers, hundreds of thousands of deaths from heart disease. Countless days of suffering can be avoided not only from cancer and heart disease but also from other ills that sound less ominous but still take their toll on our families, our work, and generally how we feel about facing each morning.

It is time for us to take an active role in our own health care. Medical costs in the last few years have risen twice as fast as inflation, hospital costs have risen at three times the rate of the consumer price index. And still we have not made a serious dent in the incidence of the leading diseases.

Some people have already set out on the high road to health—and they're getting results. Over the last decade, Americans have begun switching from butter to margarine, overcoming the obstacle of taste to lower their fat and cholesterol levels. Many are cutting down on salt, consuming fewer calories. They are exercising a bit more, and trying to get themselves exercised over stressful events a bit less. We won't be able to scientifically evaluate the effects of these changes for a while, but already we are seeing a decline in heart disease. Some gerontologists at the University of Southern California and statisticians elsewhere are even projecting that we will all be living longer by the year 2000 if current health trends continue.

From this point on, if we are to make any further inroads in reducing the major threats to our health, we will have to focus on strengthening our body's natural defense mechanisms, our immune system. In short, we will have to take steps to make ourselves as healthy as possible so we can resist disease from within rather than waiting for rescue from without. The body is very good at preserving itself if given half a chance—humans have spent millions of years evolving systems designed precisely to preserve us. And we know today how to give ourselves the best chance. The job is ours.

We can stop killing ourselves—and we can start today.

2
The Mind-Body Link and the Immune System

GREGORY WAS ten years old and all the doctors gave him six months to live. He'd had radiation treatment, but the tumor in his brain was growing bigger. They could not operate. He was terminal, they said. That was September 1978.

Then he went to the Menninger Clinic in Kansas, where the doctors tried the only possibility left—they told Gregory that he would have to try to fix his brain by using his brain.

Gregory became the Blue Leader in his fantasy, the leader of a squadron of fighter planes. He thought of his brain as the solar system and the tumor as an invading planetoid which he said was threatening to kill him.

Each night, the Blue Leader would close his eyes, breathe deeply, settle into his cockpit, and take off into the solar system to do battle. And each night, soon after takeoff, the entire squadron would zero in on the invading planetoid, fire torpedoes and laser beams—those represented the killer lymphocytes in his immune system—until gradually they blew the foe to bits.

Gregory got worse for the first few months after he began this visualization therapy, but he stuck with it. Then, eight months after he began—two months beyond the doctors' expectations—he noticed he was regaining some control over his hands, and his eye stopped troubling him. Soon after, he was able to take off the leg brace without falling down. Then his walking began to improve—he walked with greater ease than he could remember for a long time. He felt good again.

Then one night when the Blue Leader took off, for the first time he could not find his target. "Dad, it's gone," he yelled. His father calmed him down and urged him to try again. "Dad, there are only some funny white spots where the planetoid is supposed to be."

In February 1980, the Menninger Clinic's CAT scan of Gregory's brain showed that the tumor was indeed gone—the only unusual thing in the picture, according to Dr. Patricia Norris, was a cluster of bony white chips, a little calcium deposit, exactly where the tumor used to be.

The Blue Leader is gone—Gregory is with us today.

MBL—The Mind-Body Link—Past and Present

The mind and body are inseparable, inextricably bound, interdependent—they are joined, they are one. It is a marriage more permanent than any made on this earth—not in sickness or in health, not till death do they part.

It is only in the last decade that the scientific and medical communities have begun to come back around to this idea—after over three centuries in which the Cartesian mind-body split has held sway. And even today, though the realization is dawning, doctors are reluctant to encourage patients to think that their attitudes, thoughts, and emotions can play a large role in the state of their health or the progress of their illnesses.

Today we know it is so: every illness from a cold to cancer to heart disease can be affected—for better or for worse—by our moods, personalities, attitudes about whether we will get better or not. With each passing day brain researchers are learning more about how our conscious thoughts and emotions influence hormone levels, organ functions, and the most powerful weapon in the defense of our health—the immune system.

There is even a new name for this burgeoning field of research—psychoneuroimmunology—the study of the interplay of the mind, the nervous system, and the immune system. It is one of the fastest-growing fields of research, likely to be one of the most important fields of health to be pursued in the coming years.

The Power of Suggestion Gains Acceptance

The power of the mind to influence the body has been recognized for thousands of years—in practices ranging from voodoo to chicken soup "therapy" and to the magic of a mother's kiss. But this healing force has been invoked most often on the fringes of the healing profession. Only recently have scientific studies been done that demonstrate the reliable potency of these healing powers we all possess.

But we have much to learn about how to use this internal force. Even today this proof of the mind's power over the body is still disparaged as "only the placebo effect."

We Aim to Please

The placebo effect—the process whereby someone feels better and gets better without being given "real" medication—rather a sugar pill or salt solution—has been shown to help patients in an average of one-third of cases.*

Placebo, in Latin, means "I shall please." The result of taking a placebo is sometimes a belief so strong that a patient can reverse the effects of even very potent drugs. One doctor at New York Hospital tested this possibility while treating women suffering nausea in the early stages of pregnancy because their muscles were contracting abnormally. He offered a pill to soothe them—and the nausea vanished. The pill, far from an innocuous sugar tablet, was actually ipecac—one of the most powerful emetics used to induce vomiting in those who have swallowed poisons.

The women's belief, however, was stronger than the drug.

Surgery as Placebo

Some thoroughly accepted medical practices have been shown later to have worked more because people believed in them than because of any inherent healing properties of the treatment. This has been the case with treatments ranging from drugs to surgery, for even something as serious as angina, the chest pains of heart disease.

In the last two hundred years, every treatment used for angina worked for 70 to 90 percent of the patients at first, as long as the ministering physician believed in the treatment (according to two Harvard researchers who have published a review of angina treatments over that period). But as soon as some "newer" therapy came into favor, the old method dropped to only 30 to 40 percent effectiveness.

---

*In a review of fifteen placebo studies by the late Dr. Henry Beecher, then professor of anesthesiology at Harvard Medical School, a range of 15 to 58 percent of patients on placebo found relief from anything from pain to seasickness.

Even so, 30 to 40 percent effectiveness is not bad, considering that *not one of these treatments is regarded as effective today*. Not one.

Placebos have, in some cases, been shown to be as effective as surgery. In the 1950s and 1960s, when medical ethics and respect for patients' rights were not as well considered as they are today, some researchers did a study involving sham surgery and came up with stunning results. They told two groups of heart patients that they were going to undergo an operation found effective in treating angina pectoris. Only one group actually had the surgical procedure. The other group was put under anesthesia, cut open, and the incision was closed. The patients who had undergone the sham surgery did better than the ones who had the genuine operation.

Some cardiologists today are beginning to suspect that the currently popular coronary bypass operation might just fall into a similar category of doing no more than a placebo would for many patients undergoing the operation—but at considerably higher cost and risk.

Placebos can have negative effects as well—if they're accompanied by a negative suggestion. Studies have shown that people can get diarrhea, rashes, headaches, nausea, even heart palpitations when told they were receiving a powerful medication that might produce such effects. In a Japanese study, two physicians applied leaves to the skins of hypnotized subjects: if the patients were told the leaves were harmless, nothing happened; if they were told it was poison ivy, the subjects' skin actually became red and irritated.

Though the exact mechanism involved with the placebo effect is not clearly understood, most researchers agree that the patient is bringing about some biochemical change within himself or herself. A pain researcher at the University of California, San Francisco, examined a number of people who had just had their wisdom teeth extracted and were in considerable pain. He told all that they were receiving a pain reliever, but some received morphine and others received a salt solution. One-third of each group said the pain disappeared soon after the injection.

What happened? Those who were given salt water managed, by themselves—having nothing to do with the saltwater condition—to step up production of their body's natural opiate, endorphins, which can be more potent than morphine. To verify this assumption, the researcher gave the pain-free, saltwater patients a drug called naloxone, which blocks the effects of the brain's endorphins. And indeed their pain returned. In short, it seems that the placebo effect can represent our ability to control biochemical reactions in the brain.

Similarly, skin problems such as warts, which are known to be caused by viruses (and which 20 to 50 percent of Americans have at one time or another), have also been shown to be triggered by emotional upsets. And they can be eliminated through mental concentration. One study, conducted at Massachusetts General Hospital, found that in 50 percent of cases that did not respond to any other treatment, hypnosis, which is simply a form of mental concentration, proved effective in getting rid of the warts.

Attitude, Emotions Can Make Us Flourish . . . or Wither

Our attitude about ourselves can have a critical effect on how we feel and function. It determines whether we are under stress—as you'll see in chapter 5, stress is not an external event working on us but an internal series of bodily responses triggered by our perception of events and our judgment about whether or not we are comfortably in control of them.

If we harbor the fear that our lives are forever just beyond our control, then we constantly trigger the stress response within us. Stress, negative emotions such as anger and hostility, grief, anxiety, depression, can stimulate the release of hormones that damage arteries and lower the activity of lymphocytes and other elements of the immune system that fight off infectious agents. The mind can sabotage the body.

Children's physical growth can even be affected by emotional trauma. A child deprived of loving emotional support—one with abusive parents, for example, or indifferent institutional guardians—can actually stop growing. The emotional deprivation retards not only mental development but physical development as well. The condition is called "psychosocial dwarfism" and is not as uncommon as we might wish.

Psychologists have also reported cases in which young girls who were victims of incest—and who developed a great fear of growing up into even more vulnerable womanhood—have actually kept themselves from developing women's bodies. Not until they begin psychotherapy and come to grips with much of their haunting pasts do they begin—sometimes even as late as in their twenties and thirties—finally to develop breasts and hips. First they heal their minds, then their bodies.

The mind is a powerful force—the mind and body are a powerful team. The medical profession is finally facing the realization that the way we live—how happy and settled or stressful we feel—can have the greatest influence on whether we get sick or get well.

But no matter what the external reality—even if objectively you face no more hardships than other calmer individuals—if you *feel* you are under stress, your body reacts with all the chemical and physiological changes the stress response brings, including lowered immunity. Among two groups of smokers followed by a researcher at the Veterans Administration in Miami, those who perceived themselves to be under greater stress developed lung cancer, while the other smokers who did not feel themselves under much stress (but who had the same number of emotionally charged events going on in their lives, such as marriage, divorce, family illness) are still free of cancer.

In another study of healthy graduate students, those who felt themselves to be under greater stress had only one-third the other group's level of "natural killer cell activity"—white blood cells that can recognize and fight foreign cells instantly without having had to be exposed to them before, and which are vital to maintaining good health.

The Future for Our Minds, Our Bodies

The challenge now—for the medical profession and for us all—is to start taking advantage of the placebo effect, the power of mind over body, to help make us healthy and keep us that way.

No one is suggesting that we abandon the advances made so far in the world of traditional medicine. We would be in a sorry state without the magnificent vaccines that dedicated scientists have cultured and refined, and we'd be fools if we turned our backs on antibiotics when we contract bacterial infections.

But we would be equally foolish to ignore this other powerful resource that we carry around on our shoulders all our lives.

Scientists are already working with animals, training them to suppress and activate their immune response at will. At the University of Rochester, researchers have trained animals to suppress their immune responses just as Pavlov taught his dogs to slobber at the sound of a bell. First the animals were given, along with some saccharin, a drug that suppresses the immune system. After a while, the lab animals connected the immunosuppressant drug and saccharin so strongly that when they were given the saccharin without the immunosuppressant drug, they lowered their immune response anyway, by themselves.

Suppressing the immune system by limiting the body's production of antibodies is usually not desirable for staying healthy. However, it can be helpful in those conditions in which the immune system over-reacts—as it does in hay fever and other allergic responses, lupus, rheumatoid arthritis, and ulcerative colitis, to name a few.

Even more important is the implication that we can learn to acti-vate the immune system as easily as suppress it—just as Gregory did in fighting his brain tumor. And it is likely to be this ability to stimulate our natural immunity that will provide the most significant future breakthroughs in our fight against nearly every illness, from colds to AIDS (acquired immune deficiency syndrome) to the many intractable forms of cancer.

Most of us forget that even the drugs we use now—vaccines, antibi-otics, the chemotherapy in cancer treatments—work only insofar as they boost our immunity. They cannot work without the immune sys-tem. Vaccines merely trigger our immune response in advance to give us a head start when a virus tries to settle in. Antibiotics kill only some of the invading fungi or bacteria; but for us to recover from even the most minor infection, we must kill every single bacterium—not one can escape or it will multiply and take over. And that job falls to our granulocytes (white blood cells), to our antibodies, to properdin, to complement (the collective name for the nine proteins that blow bacte-rial cells wide open), to macrophages and to our lymphocytes—all of which are parts of our complex immune response.

Chemotherapy, too, can kill only a small portion of the cancer cells. It is our own killer T-lymphocytes in the immune system that must do the rest if we are to survive.

Certain small but very important steps can lead us toward en-hanced immunity and better health. We can learn to modify our diet, exercise, and change daily habits, including how we respond emo-tionally under stress.

The time has come for us to take advantage of this dawning awareness of the mind-body link.

How Healthy
Are You?

WHERE DO YOU STAND right now, what risks do you face, if you keep on living as you do? Take a test to compute your body's *real* age and find out if your habits are making you old before your time.

3
Health Test— Compute Your Body's *Real* Age

WHEN PEOPLE ASK how old we are, we usually respond with the number of years that have passed since our birth. But that doesn't tell the whole story.

Our real age—the age that lets us know how close we're coming to the edge of night—depends upon how we spend our days. The current life expectancy for men is about seventy-one, for women, about seventy-eight. Each of us secretly believes that those averages apply to someone else: we, of course, are the exceptions. Well, we can be exceptions—and we can rewrite the odds. Some gerontologists estimate that if health habits continue to improve, men and women may live four and eight years longer by the year 2000. But it won't be an accident of genes that keeps us going—it will be very deliberate changes in how we live.

This test will help you see in round numbers whether you're making yourself old or young for your age and how your chronological age compares to your real *health age*. And it should help you pinpoint which habits to pursue and which to squelch if you want to stop killing yourself. Draw two columns on a piece of paper, one marked ADD and the other, SUBTRACT, and keep score.

1. I am married.   *Subtract 3.*
   I am separated, divorced or widowed.   *Add 3.*
   I am single and over 30.   *Add 1.* Under 30.   *Add 0.*
2. I never have smoked.   *Subtract 2.*
   I quit smoking over 10 years ago.   *Add 0.*
   I quit smoking within the last ten years.   *Add 2.*

I smoke 10 cigarettes a day, or an occasional pipe or cigar. *Add 6.*

I smoke 20 or more cigarettes a day, or regularly smoke a pipe or cigar.   *Add 12.*

I smoke 40 cigarettes a day.   *Add 16.*

I smoke more than 40 cigarettes.   *Add 20.*

3. I would say that I am basically happy with my life.   *Subtract 4.*

I am not terribly happy about how my life is going.   *Add 3.*

Most days, I am very troubled and unhappy about how my life is going.   *Add 5.*

4. I eat red meat at least once and often twice a day, use butter but never margarine, and eat fried foods often.   *Add 6.*

I eat red meat 4 to 7 times a week, use both butter and margarine, and occasionally eat fried foods.   *Add 4.*

I eat red meat less than 4 times a week and eat fish or chicken instead, use very little butter or margarine, rarely eat fried foods.   *Subtract 3.*

5. I eat both fresh fruits and vegetables twice a day.   *Subtract 4.*

I eat both fresh fruits and vegetables once a day.   *Subtract 3.*

I eat either a piece of fruit or a vegetable once a day. *Subtract 1.*

I eat fruits or vegetables less than 5 times a week.   *Add 1.*

I eat fruits or vegetables less than once a week.   *Add 3.*

6. I enjoy my work and find the environment and my colleagues stimulating.   *Subtract 4.*

I enjoy my work most of the time, but there are often seriously aggravating problems that arise.   *Subtract 1.*

I do not look forward to going in to work and feel great relief when the day is over and I can get out of there.   *Add 4.*

7. I do not drive a car, or drive less than 5000 miles a year. *Subtract 5.*

I drive less than 10,000 miles a year.   *Subtract 4.*

I drive more than 25,000 miles a year.   *Add 5.*

8. I rarely wear a seat belt when I am in a car.   *Add 5.*

I wear a seat belt more than half the time in a car.   *Add 2.*

I always wear a seat belt.   *Subtract 1.*

9. I never feel like I've gotten enough sleep.   *Add 3.*

I often wake up wishing I could get a little more sleep.   *Add 2.*

I usually wake up feeling refreshed.   *Subtract 2.*

10. I am very overweight (more than 20 percent above my ideal weight).   *Add 5.*

    I am slightly overweight and could stand to lose at least 15 pounds.   *Add 3.*

    I am about at my ideal weight, give or take a few pounds. *Add 0.*

    I am underweight (more than 15 percent below my ideal weight).   *Add 3.*

11. I drink more than 3 alcoholic beverages a day (a bottle of beer, glass of wine, or 2 ounces of 80 proof alcohol equals 1 drink).   *Add 5.*

    I drink more than 14 alcoholic beverages a week.   *Add 3.*

    I drink 7 or fewer alcoholic beverages a week.   *Subtract 1.*

    I do not drink at all.   *Add 0.*

12. I smoke marijuana or take other drugs more than twice a week.   *Add 6.*

    I smoke marijuana or use other drugs once a month.   *Add 3.*

    I smoke marijuana a couple of times a year.   *Add 1.*

    I never take drugs.   *Add 0.*

13. I have high or elevated blood pressure (and am under 45). *Add 4.*

    I have elevated blood pressure (and am over 45).   *Add 2.*

    My blood pressure is normal.   *Add 0.*

14. My father or mother had heart disease or cancer before age 60.   *Add 2.*

    My father or mother had heart disease or cancer after age 60.   *Add 0.*

15. I have diabetes.   *Add 5.* (If not, add 0.)

16. I engage in vigorous exercise for at least 30 minutes 3 times a week.   *Subtract 10.*

    I engage in vigorous exercise for at least 30 minutes twice a week.   *Subtract 5.*

    I exercise regularly daily, although it is not a strenuous aerobic workout.   *Subtract 4.*

    I exercise less than once a week.   *Add 2.*

    I work at a desk, rarely exercise.   *Add 10.*

17. I have had more than three colds or infections in the last year.   *Add 3.*

    I have had 1 to 3 colds or infections in the last year.   *Add 1.*

    I have had no colds or infections in the last year.   *Subtract 3.*

18. I never feel as if there is enough time in the day to get every-thing that I've scheduled done; I feel constantly under stress.   *Add 6.*

    I often feel as if I must hurry up to get everything done; I often feel under great stress.   *Add 3.*

    I occasionally feel as if there are not enough hours in the day, but I usually do not let it upset me.   *Add 0.*

    I schedule my days so I get done most of what I've planned; and if I don't finish, it doesn't worry me at all. Tomorrow's another day.   *Subtract 6.*

19. I have quite a temper; and it especially makes me angry to have to wait in line and waste my time.   *Add 5.*

    I get angry occasionally, but I don't sit and stew about it or hold a grudge.   *Add 0.*

    I get angry sometimes, but it never lasts long and most of the time I realize later it was a silly thing even to bother about.   *Subtract 3.*

    I never get angry; at least I never show it. I don't think it's right to show anger or other intense emotions either.   *Add 2.*

20. When I get tense, I try to use stress-reduction techniques to calm down.   *Subtract 5.*

    When I get tense, I don't take any special action; I just hope I'll unwind after a while.   *Add 5.*

Your Score

Add up the numbers in the add column. Then add up the numbers in the subtract column. Find the difference between them.

For example, if you have 32 in the add column and 20 in the subtract column, then the difference is 12. (If the numbers in the columns were reversed, the difference would be -12.)

Now you take the difference you have just computed and divide that number by 6. In the above example you'd divide 12 (or -12) by 6 and get 2 or (-2).

Now either add or subtract that number (if the add column came to a higher total, then add; if the subtract column was higher, then sub-tract) from your age. That gives you your real health age. In the above example, the person wound up 2 years older (or in the reverse case 2 years younger) than his chronological age.

How to Get Better

No matter what your score, if you turned out younger or older than your years, go back through the test and see how you could be doing even better—see which questions brought down your health score. Perhaps the exercise question really held back your chances at longer life, or maybe it was the smoking, or the diet question. You can do something about these health habits.

If your results don't seem dramatic—say, you only came out to be a few years younger or older than your years, bear this in mind: the ill effects of bad habits grow as you age. If you are only in your thirties and your habits are already making you a couple of years older than you are, then it is possible that by the time you reach your forties, the cumulative effects of those habits could be shaving twice that many years off your life, and by the next decade, they'll take off eight years of your life, and by the next decade—if there is one—you may be as much as sixteen years older than you could and should be.

Even more important to keep in mind is that poor health habits don't just kill you suddenly—they can make your life miserable for many years beforehand as well. And what you're after—what we're all after, and what this book aims to help you achieve—is a healthy, vigorous, happy life for as many years as you have in this world.

4
Discover Your Risks

Face the Music—and Keep on Dancing

THE FIRST STEP you must take in becoming master of your fate is knowing what possible risks you face. Risks vary according to many factors, the most obvious being age, sex, and race. A boy under twenty is most likely to die of a car accident, while a man over thirty-five better be on the alert for a heart attack and a woman of that same age should know the early-warning signs for breast cancer.

The tables let you see into a possible future—the diseases and disasters that you may face in the next ten years—if you don't take any special preventive action. But bear in mind that they are, after all, just average statistics. And humans are much cleverer than statistics. If you put your mind to it, and throw in a little body action as well, you can change habits in daily life that can do more to save your life—or kill you—than those factors of age, sex, and race that you cannot change.

Risk Highlights

For those who are instantly afflicted with the dread disease MEGO (My Eyes Glaze Over) when faced with tables and charts, here is an overview of your possible future health picture. It is important to bear in mind that you face two kinds of risks: the immediate, short-term, *right now* risks; and those that won't catch up with you until later, but they'll come *soon enough* unless you take action.

Age 1-20

RIGHT NOW RISKS

Accidents. The major risk is highway accidents, accounting for nearly half of all deaths in this age group. Drownings, burns, falls, and poisonings account for the remaining accidental deaths. Boys face a special risk of firearm accidents.

Suicide and homicide. The suicide rate for teenagers is rising dramatically. Noticing the symptoms of depression early can help. Blacks of this age are especially at risk for homicide—carrying weapons is one of the factors that increases the chances of getting killed.

SOON ENOUGH

Heart disease. The exercise and diet habits that begin in childhood, making for inactive, overweight youngsters, can carry through to adulthood, making for heavy adults who are at high risk.

Tooth and gum problems. Again diet and hygiene habits get set young. Though not life-threatening, tooth problems can certainly affect the quality of one's daily life for a long time.

Age 20 to 35

RIGHT NOW RISKS

Accidents, murder, and suicide. These three account for the majority of all deaths.

Homicide and suicide. There are twice as many murders as there were in the 1950s, nearly three times as many suicides. Blacks are more at risk for homicide than whites, despite the fact that homicide rates among blacks have been declining since the mid-1970s; whites are more at risk for suicide; and males of both races have about three times the risk of dying as females.

Heart disease and cancer. Stroke, along with heart disease and breast and cervical cancer, are starting to make their presence felt even this early.

SOON ENOUGH

Lung and cervical cancer, and variations on heart disease. Smoking among younger women is going up. In the sixties, girls smoked at half the rate of boys; now they puff at about equal rates. About 20 to 30 percent of children under eighteen smoke regularly. So by the time they reach this age group, many have been smoking for over fifteen years.

Age 36 to 50

RIGHT NOW RISKS

Heart disease and stroke. After age forty, heart disease becomes the number one killer for all age groups. Men are three times as likely to die of heart disease as women; blacks are at much higher risk of strokes than whites.

Accidents. For men, car accidents remain a constant threat. The incidence went down for a while between 1973 and 1976 (when the oil shortage was the most severe and driving speeds hit an all-time low), but it has begun to rise again.

Cancer. Cancer deaths, primarily from lung cancer, have begun rising since 1950. Breast cancer for women and lung cancer for men are the leading threats.

SOON ENOUGH

Cirrhosis of the liver. It is actually a present danger for this age group, but will soon become an even greater risk.

Heart disease and cancer. If not present already, it may be a matter of time.

Diabetes and arthritis. The eating, smoking and exercise habits of a half century may soon catch up.

Age 51 to 65

RIGHT NOW RISKS

Heart disease, cancer, and stroke. These are the leading causes of death. Men are three times as likely to die of heart disease as women. Cancer and stroke seem to be equal-opportunity diseases when it comes to gender—though they strike in blacks at a higher rate than in whites.

Cirrhosis of the liver. The death rate doubled from 1950 to 1970, but it is now coming down slightly. Whites of both sexes are more at risk than blacks.

SOON ENOUGH

Accidents. Falls become problems later on because of increasing bone brittleness that begins for both sexes now—for women, after menopause. Exercise (and diet) can reduce this problem, as well as other circulatory, joint and back problems, that become more common.

Age 66 and over

RIGHT NOW RISKS

Heart disease, cancer, and stroke. These account for 75 percent of the deaths.

Accidents. Falls can be serious, though rarely directly fatal.

Arthritis. Forty-four percent of people over 65 suffer arthritis—more than twice as many as those with heart disease. While this painful condition accounts for few deaths, it causes people to spend nearly as many days in bed as heart disease does.

The stress of retirement, bringing with it dramatic changes in one's status and financial situation, as well as seeing one's friends begin to die, can be a major contributor to the ailments at this age. Right now, 80 percent of people in this age group suffer from one or more chronic conditions. But this need not be. Being aged does not have to mean disability or suffering. Even if some of the conditions discussed above do emerge, individuals who have been taking steps to stay healthy all along can usually cope with the least discomfort.

Find Your Risks

The following table shows the ten most pressing risks you'll face—things that can kill you—at any point from now through the next ten years, at whatever age you are. The ailments and conditions are the top ten causes of death for the age groups listed, ranked from highest to lowest.

The ranking is based on an averaging of mortality statistics. If you have a special family history or personal habits that predispose you to a certain disease, then, for you, that disease might move up higher in the rankings. It can also move lower, if your habits protect you.

Once you find which problems you may be facing, turn to the end of this chapter for a summary of the factors that put you at risk for each disease. Then turn to the appropriate chapter for a complete explanation of what you're doing daily to put you at risk—and how you can reduce those risks and increase your chances for a long, healthy life.

RISK TABLE

Age	Rank	White Male	White Female	Black Male	Black Female
5 to 9	1	Motor vehicle accidents	Motor vehicle accidents	Motor vehicle accidents	Motor vehicle accidents
	2	Drownings	Leukemia	Drownings	Fires
	3	Leukemia	Fires	Fires	Homicide
	4	Firearm accidents	Brain cancer	Homicide	Drownings
	5	Fires	Drownings	Leukemia	Circulatory birth defects
	6	Brain Cancer	Circulatory birth defects	Firearm accidents	Pneumonia
	7	Circulatory birth defects	Pneumonia	Circulatory birth defects	Leukemia
	8	Machine-related accidents	Homicide	Brain cancer	Brain cancer
	9	Homicide	Cystic fibrosis	Pneumonia	Hydrocephalus
	10	Suicide	Infantile paralysis	Falls	Anemias
10 to 14	1	Motor vehicle accidents	Motor vehicle accidents	Homicide	Homicide
	2	Suicide	Homicide	Motor vehicle accidents	Motor vehicle accidents
	3	Drownings	Suicide	Drownings	Drownings
	4	Homicide	Leukemia	Suicide	Fires
	5	Firearm accidents	Fires	Firearm accidents	Leukemia
	6	Leukemia	Brain cancer	Fires	Suicide
	7	Machine-related accidents	Pneumonia	Pneumonia	Pneumonia
	8	Poisonings	Circulatory birth defects	Leukemia	Anemias
	9	Falls	Drownings	Machine-related accidents	Circulatory birth defects
	10	Circulatory birth defects	Poisonings	Epilepsy	Poisonings

Age	Rank	White Male	White Female	Black Male	Black Female
15 to 19	1	Motor vehicle accidents	Motor vehicle accidents	Homicide	Homicide
	2	Suicide	Suicide	Motor vehicle accidents	Motor vehicle accidents
	3	Homicide	Homicide	Drownings	Suicide
	4	Drownings	Poisonings	Suicide	Poisonings
	5	Poisonings	Leukemia	Poisonings	Strokes, blood vessel disorders
	6	Machine-related accidents	Fires	Firearm accidents	Fires
	7	Firearm accidents	Strokes, blood vessel disorders	Fires	Leukemia
	8	Falls	Pneumonia	Pneumonia	Pneumonia
	9	Leukemia	Circulatory birth defects	Machine-related accidents	Anemias
	10	Electrocution	Drownings	Epilepsy	Drownings
20 to 24	1	Motor vehicle accidents	Motor vehicle accidents	Homicide	Homicide
	2	Suicide	Suicide	Motor vehicle accidents	Motor vehicle accidents
	3	Homicide	Homicide	Suicide	Suicide
	4	Poisonings	Strokes, blood vessel disorders	Drownings	Strokes, blood vessel disorders
	5	Drownings	Poisonings	Poisonings	Cirrhosis
	6	Machine-related accidents	Leukemia	Cirrhosis	Poisonings
	7	Falls	Pneumonia	Heart disease	Pneumonia
	8	Aircraft accidents	Hodgkin's disease	Pneumonia	Fires

	Col 1	Col 2	Col 3	Col 4
9	Fires	Fires	Fires	Heart disease
10	Electrocution	Breast cancer	Strokes, blood vessel disorders	Leukemia
25 to 29				
1	Motor vehicle accidents	Motor vehicle accidents	Homicide	Homicide
2	Suicide	Suicide	Motor vehicle accidents	Cirrhosis
3	Homicide	Homicide	Suicide	Motor Vehicle accidents
4	Heart disease	Breast cancer	Cirrhosis	Strokes, blood vessel disorders
5	Poisonings	Strokes, blood vessel disorders	Heart disease	Suicide
6	Drownings	Leukemia	Drownings	Breast cancer
7	Machine-related accidents	Poisonings	Poisonings	Heart disease
8	Cirrhosis	Heart disease	Strokes, blood vessel disorders	Pneumonia
9	Aircraft accidents	Cirrhosis	Pneumonia	Poisonings
10	Vascular lesions	Cervical cancer	Alcoholism	Cervical cancer
30 to 34				
1	Motor vehicle accidents	Suicide	Homicide	Homicide
2	Suicide	Motor vehicle accidents	Heart disease	Cirrhosis
3	Heart disease	Breast cancer	Motor vehicle accidents	Heart disease
4	Homicide	Strokes, blood vessel disorders	Cirrhosis	Strokes, blood vessel disorders
5	Cirrhosis	Heart disease	Strokes, blood vessel disorders	Breast cancer

Age	Rank	White Male	White Female	Black Male	Black Female
30 to 34	6	Vascular lesions	Homicide	Suicide	Motor vehicle accidents
	7	Lung cancer	Cirrhosis	Alcoholism	Cervical cancer
	8	Machine-related accidents	Cervical cancer	Pneumonia	Pneumonia
	9	Poisonings	Lung cancer	Drownings	Suicide
	10	Aircraft accidents	Leukemia	Poisonings	Diabetes
35 to 39	1	Heart disease	Breast cancer	Homicide	Heart disease
	2	Motor vehicle accidents	Arteriosclerotic heart disease	Heart disease	Cirrhosis
	3	Suicide	Suicide	Cirrhosis	Strokes, blood vessel disorders
	4	Cirrhosis	Motor vehicle accidents	Motor vehicle accidents	Breast cancer
	5	Homicide	Strokes, blood vessel disorders	Strokes, blood vessel disorders	Homicide
	6	Lung cancer	Cirrhosis	Lung cancer	Lung cancer
	7	Strokes, blood vessel disorders	Lung cancer	Alcoholism	Cervical cancer
	8	Machine-related accidents	Homicide	Pneumonia	Motor vehicle accidents
	9	Intestinal-rectal cancer	Intestinal-rectal cancer	Suicide	Pneumonia
	10	Pneumonia	Cervical cancer	Diabetes	Diabetes

40 to 44	1	Heart disease	Breast cancer	Heart disease	Heart disease
	2	Lung cancer	Heart disease	Homicide	Strokes, blood vessel disorders
	3	Cirrhosis	Lung cancer	Cirrhosis	Cirrhosis
	4	Motor vehicle accidents	Strokes, blood vessel disorders	Lung cancer	Breast cancer
	5	Suicide	Cirrhosis	Strokes, blood vessel disorders	Lung cancer
	6	Vascular lesions	Suicide	Motor vehicle accidents	Cervical cancer
	7	Homicide	Motor vehicle accidents	Pneumonia	Homicide
	8	Intestinal-rectal cancer	Intestinal-rectal cancer	Alcoholism	Diabetes
	9	Pneumonia	Ovarian cancer	Cancer of esophagus	Pneumonia
	10	Alcoholism	Cervical cancer	Diabetes	Heart disease
45 to 49	1	Heart disease	Heart disease	Heart disease	Heart disease
	2	Lung cancer	Breast cancer	Lung cancer	Strokes, blood vessel disorders
	3	Cirrhosis	Lung cancer	Cirrhosis	Breast cancer
	4	Suicide	Strokes, blood vessel disorders	Strokes, blood vessel disorders	Cirrhosis
	5	Motor vehicle accidents	Cirrhosis	Homicide	Lung cancer
	6	Strokes, blood vessel disorders	Intestinal-rectal cancer	Pneumonia	Diabetes
	7	Intestinal-rectal cancer	Ovarian cancer	Motor vehicle accidents	Cervical cancer
	8	Homicide	Suicide	Alcoholism	Intestinal-rectal cancer
	9	Pneumonia	Motor vehicle accidents	Cancer of esophagus	Heart disease
	10	Diabetes	Diabetes	Diabetes	Pneumonia

Age	Rank	White Male	White Female	Black Male	Black Female
50 to 54	1	Heart disease	Heart disease	Heart disease	Heart disease
	2	Lung cancer	Breast cancer	Lung cancer	Strokes, blood vessel disorders
	3	Cirrhosis	Lung cancer	Strokes, blood vessel disorders	Breast cancer
	4	Strokes, blood vessel disorders	Strokes, blood vessel disorders	Cirrhosis	Lung cancer
	5	Intestinal-rectal cancer	Intestinal-rectal cancer	Homicide	Diabetes
	6	Suicide	Cirrhosis	Pneumonia	Cirrhosis
	7	Motor vehicle accidents	Ovarian cancer	Cancer of esophagus	Intestinal-rectal cancer
	8	Diabetes	Suicide	Motor vehicle accidents	Cervical cancer
	9	Pneumonia	Diabetes	Intestinal-rectal cancer	Heart disease
	10	Bronchitis and emphysema	Motor vehicle accidents	Alcoholism	Pneumonia
55 to 59	1	Heart disease	Heart disease	Heart disease	Heart disease
	2	Lung cancer	Breast cancer	Lung cancer	Strokes, blood vessel disorders
	3	Strokes, blood vessel disorders	Lung cancer	Strokes, blood vessel disorders	Breast cancer
	4	Cirrhosis	Strokes, blood vessel disorders	Cirrhosis	Diabetes

	Column 1	Column 2	Column 3	Column 4
5	Intestinal-rectal cancer	Intestinal-rectal cancer	Pneumonia	Lung cancer
6	Suicide	Ovarian cancer	Intestinal-rectal cancer	Intestinal-rectal cancer
7	Bronchitis and emphysema	Cirrhosis	Prostate cancer	Cirrhosis
8	Pneumonia	Diabetes	Cancer of esophagus	Hypertensive heart disease
9	Motor vehicle accidents	Rheumatic heart disease	Homicide	Cervical cancer
10	Diabetes	Pneumonia	Diabetes	Strokes, blood vessel disorders
60 to 64				
1	Heart disease	Heart disease	Heart disease	Heart disease
2	Lung cancer	Strokes, blood vessel disorders	Lung cancer	Strokes, blood vessel disorders
3	Strokes, blood vessel disorders	Breast cancer	Strokes, blood vessel disorders	Diabetes
4	Intestinal-rectal cancer	Lung cancer	Prostate cancer	Breast cancer
5	Cirrhosis	Intestinal-rectal cancer	Pneumonia	Intestinal-rectal cancer
6	Bronchitis and emphysema	Diabetes	Intestinal-rectal cancer	Lung cancer
7	Diseases of arteries	Ovarian cancer	Diabetes	Hypertensive heart disease
8	Prostate cancer	Cirrhosis	Cirrhosis	Pneumonia
9	Pneumonia	Rheumatic heart disease	Cancer of esophagus	Cirrhosis
10	Diabetes	Pneumonia	Stomach cancer	Kidney disease

Age	Rank	White Male	White Female	Black Male	Black Female
65 to 69	1	Heart disease	Heart disease	Heart disease	Heart disease
	2	Lung cancer	Strokes, blood vessel disorders	Strokes, blood vessel disorders	Strokes, blood vessel disorders
	3	Strokes, blood vessel disorders	Breast cancer	Lung cancer	Diabetes
	4	Intestinal-rectal cancer	Intestinal-rectal cancer	Prostate cancer	Intestinal-rectal cancer
	5	Bronchitis and emphysema	Lung cancer	Pneumonia	Breast cancer
	6	Prostate cancer	Diabetes	Intestinal-rectal cancer	Hypertensive heart disease
	7	Diseases of arteries	Ovarian cancer	Diabetes	Lung cancer
	8	Pneumonia	Pneumonia	Hypertensive heart disease	Pneumonia
	9	Cirrhosis	Diseases of arteries	Stomach cancer	Diseases of arteries
	10	Diabetes	Cirrhosis	Diseases of arteries	Uterine cancer
70 to 74	1	Heart disease	Heart disease	Heart disease	Heart disease
	2	Strokes, blood vessel disorders	Strokes, blood vessel disorders	Strokes, blood vessel disorders	Strokes, blood vessel disorders
	3	Lung cancer	Intestinal-rectal cancer	Lung cancer	Diabetes
	4	Intestinal-rectal cancer	Breast cancer	Prostate cancer	Intestinal-rectal cancer
	5	Prostate cancer	Diabetes	Pneumonia	Breast cancer
	6	Diseases of arteries	Lung cancer	Intestinal-rectal cancer	Hypertensive heart disease

7	Pneumonia	Pneumonia	Diabetes	Diseases of arteries
8	Bronchitis and emphysema	Diseases of arteries	Diseases of arteries	Pneumonia
9	Diabetes	Ovarian cancer	Hypertensive heart disease	Lung cancer
10	Stomach cancer	Hypertensive heart disease	Stomach cancer	Kidney disease

Reprinted with the permission of Prospective Medicine Center, Indiana, from *Prospective Medicine* by Jack H. Hall, M.D., and Jack D. Zwemer, D.D.S., Ph.D., copyright © 1979 by Methodist Hospital of Indiana.

Brief Summary of Risk Factors for Various Diseases

Here is a brief sketch of which habits and conditions put you at the greatest risk for developing these major disorders. You'll find far more detail in later chapters on the role these risk factors play.

Cancer. High-fat, low-fiber diet, smoking, attitude, family history.

Car accidents. Drinking alcohol, not wearing seat belts, taking drugs (especially tranquilizers or sedatives), mileage (the more, the greater the risk).

Cirrhosis of the liver. Drinking alcohol to excess (more than twenty-five drinks per week).

Diabetes. Weight, diet, exercise, family history.

Emphysema and bronchitis. Smoking.

Heart disease. Smoking, little exercise, being overweight, high-fat, low-fiber diet, Type A personality, family history, elevated blood pressure, high cholesterol levels, diabetes, inability to handle stress.

Homicide. Arrest record—a history of crimes involving violence or the threat of it, use of weapons.

Pneumonia. Drinking, history of past pneumonia, smoking, emphysema.

Suicide. Depression, characterized by crying fits or inability to cry, withdrawal, disturbances in appetite, sleep, energy, and concentration, overwhelming anxiety, fear, guilt, pessimism, and possibly an increase in drug or alcohol use.

Stroke. Smoking, cholesterol levels, blood pressure, exercise, diet, diabetes.

The Big Risks— Fighting the Leading Killers and Cripplers

YOU DON'T CATCH THESE major killers and cripplers like colds. For most of us, they build over years. Learn how these diseases and disasters begin and what we can do with diet, exercise, attitude, and daily habits to prevent them.

5
Stress

YOU'VE HAD A ROUGH DAY. You woke up ten minutes late and had to race to a meeting. People at the office are working as if they swallowed molasses. The boss expects this big project to be finished at the end of the week. And no one's going to appreciate how hard you've had to slog away, least of all your spouse—it's going to mean more late nights this week, frozen dinners, frayed tempers. What does it all lead to?

Stress?

Yes.

Death?

Not on your life.

Stress is not a disease. And it does not have to be harmful. But the ravages of the stress response have been linked to most of the leading killers and cripplers of our day—heart disease, cancer, diabetes, accidental injuries, suicide, cirrhosis of the liver. Feeling under stress can make us more susceptible to tuberculosis, multiple sclerosis, migraine, lower back pain, renal failure, recurrent flare-ups of herpes, even skin blemishes.

But it isn't *stress* that is killing us—it is ourselves.

There is a great deal of misunderstanding about what stress is and how best to cope with it. The latest research has turned upside down the prevailing wisdom about who exactly is most at risk—right now the wrong people are worrying about stress. And even those genuinely at risk often seek the wrong way of handling it. A multimillion-dollar antistress industry has grown up to combat a phantom disease. Over 70 million tranquilizer prescriptions are issued a year, and expensive gadgetry and stress-management counselors abound, most mistakenly teaching people to flee from stress.

You cannot flee. Stress is not an event, *out there,* coiled and ready to spring like a snake. It is a series of responses within us that is triggered not so much by a situation as by our perception of it. The predicament may not even exist—it may be the mere expectation or image of it that sets us off, heart pounding, hormones racing.

What is only beginning to be recognized is that stress is simply a part of life. It can be a destructive or an immensely productive part of life, depending upon how it is used. If you can channel it instead of avoiding it, take pleasure in your successes, eat foods that enhance your ability to cope, and learn the early-warning symptoms of stress overload, and the techniques to reverse overload when it looms, then you can be healthier than those who avoid conflict and competition altogether. You may find, as researchers are discovering, that stress can actually be good for you.

Are You at Risk?

So who should worry? Test yourself to see how you're doing in handling stress.

Are You Prone to Stress?

In this test, score as follows unless another scoring procedure is specified in the question:

4 Agree with strongly or applies nearly all the time.
3 Agree mildly or applies sometimes.
2 Agree occasionally or applies occasionally.
1 Disagree or rarely applies.
0 Disagree strongly or almost never applies.

1. When someone does something nice for me out of the blue, I wonder what he or she is really after.
2. I eat breakfast and at least one other fully-balanced meal a day. Yes, daily—0; Most days—2; Hardly ever—4.
3. Waiting in line or waiting for other people who are late really annoys me.

4. If I feel tense at the end of the day, I use deep breathing or other stress-reduction techniques to relax: Often—0; Occasionally—1; Rarely—3.
5. I often find myself having heated arguments with people close to me.
6. I have been divorced or separated recently: Yes—4; No—0.
7. I don't show my anger about everything that makes me mad, but when I blow, I blow up.
8. I have trouble falling asleep and getting up feeling refreshed.
9. I feel as if I'm wasting time if I'm not working on at least two things at once.
10. I have a network of friends who are important to me: Yes—0; No—4.
11. I do not look forward to going into work every day.
12. Most people I know would bend the truth a little if it helped them get ahead.
13. I have had more than three colds or bouts with other illnesses within the last year: Yes—4; No—0.
14. There's never enough time to do everything you want to do in life unless you really hurry up.
15. I work out strenuously for at least 15 minutes 3 times a week: Yes—0; No—4.
16. Someone very close to me has died in the last year: Yes—4; No—0.
17. I smoke per day: More than a pack—4; Less than a pack (or a pipe or cigar)—2; Nothing—0.
18. I drink the equivalent of 3 alcoholic drinks a day: Yes—2; Less—0; More—4.
19. I play to win at work and in sports—otherwise why bother?
20. I take time out for myself every day—even if it is only five minutes—to relax or think private thoughts totally uninterrupted: Yes—0; No—4.
21. I eat both fruits and vegetables at least once a day and resist eating junk food: Every day—0; Most days—2; Rarely—4.
22. I believe that nobody does something for nothing—anyone who helps you out will expect something in return.
23. I fly off the handle easily.
24. I am not very happy in my job and I'd really like to get out of it.
25. There is at least one steady person in my life whom I love, and who loves me and helps me live through the daily struggles of life: Yes—0; No—4.

Your Score

Over 80—You are dangerously prone to stress and at risk for stress-related problems—it's time for a change.

60–79—You are seriously prone to stress—learning some stress-management techniques will lower your risk.

29–59—You are about average in your experience of stress—but you can still afford to relax a bit.

Under 28—You are fairly relaxed and not likely at much risk for stress-linked problems right now—so help a tense friend.

Who Gets Hurt by Stress?

While it is true that our impulse to fight or take flight in the face of danger is a primitive instinct inherited from our cave-dwelling ancestors, that does not mean the reaction is automatic and beyond our control. It is our perception of ourselves and how well we are doing in our environment that influences whether we will be hurt by stress. It is not the pressures of decision making that trigger bad stress but the feeling that one's decisions are ignored, that life is overwhelming and beyond personal control.

The people making the decisions, the high-powered, high-pressured executives, who many have believed to be most vulnerable, turn out not to be. They don't rise to the top because they are genetically more equipped to handle stress. They rise because they derive healthful satisfaction from knowing that their actions count—and that seems to defuse much of the wear and tear of stress. Despite the fact that most companies buy stress-counseling services only for their top executives, it is actually their underlings who are at far greater risk.

Secretaries, along with assembly-line workers, even many middle managers, are at greater risk from stress than their bosses because all their decisions are made for them—when to start work, when to stop, how to do what they do. They fear that they can be easily replaced; they see themselves as powerless victims. And that produces bad stress.

As one cigar-chomping executive in an old cartoon put it so succinctly: "I don't get ulcers, I give them."

High-Stress Jobs

While it is more how we feel about our job rather than the job itself that determines how much stress we experience, still some occupations are more inherently stress-provoking than others.

The highest-stress jobs are those that make a lot of demands upon the person while at the same time giving the person little control over how to carry out the demands. Holding the following high-stress jobs can be as damaging to your health as smoking or having high cholesterol if you take no corrective stress-relief action: sales clerks, cashiers, waiters and waitresses, telephone operators, cooks, nurse's aides and orderlies, freight handlers, mail workers, garment stitchers, assembly-line personnel.*

However, you do not have to accept your risk even if you find yourself in one of these jobs. You may just have to work a little harder at first to control stress. In the end it is not so much what you do as how you feel about what you do that can make you flourish or crumble under stress. A florist can feel as if he is under as much debilitating strain as a Wall Street stockbroker; and if he feels under chronic pressure, his body is responding with all the stress hormones and all their accompanying dangers.

Three Kinds of Stress

Stress is not one response. Researchers have come to believe that there are actually three kinds of stress: normal stress, distress or bad stress (which is normal stress that has become chronic), and eustress or good stress. While the three stress responses follow similar patterns, they are not identical in their effects on the body as was once believed.

The normal stress response is triggered by our perception or expectation of circumstances that we feel call for some kind of action from us. The stress response is what enables us to meet the challenge, adapt to change. Since life involves constant change, such reactions are obviously important: without them we cannot survive.

Imagine, for a moment, that you are walking along a dark, lonely city street and you suddenly hear heavy footsteps behind you. Here is

*According to research by Dr. Robert Karasek, assistant professor at Columbia University.

what is going on in your body—the three-stage series of the normal stress response:

The first stage is alarm. The endocrine glands release hormones, including epinephrine (adrenaline); the heartbeat speeds up, as does breathing; oxygen-rich blood is directed away from the skin to the brain and skeletal muscles for fast action. Pupils dilate to take in more information, hearing sharpens. Other hormones entering the blood increase the speed of coagulation in case of injury; muscles everywhere tense in readiness—even the scalp tightens (in animals this can make their hair stand on end); digestion slows so as not to divert any of the body's energy away from fighting or fleeing. The surge of energy, concentration, and power that comes with the stress alarm enables people to perform in crisis—sometimes astonishingly beyond their normal physical capacities.

Once the alarm stage of stress passes, and you have handled the threat—the approaching footsteps finally pass you and continue off in a different direction—the body enters the second phase, relief and recuperation. This is the point at which one can say "Whew." And the body can begin to repair any damage caused by the demands of the fight-or-flight response.

The third stage is a return to the body's normal state of relaxed alertness.

A diagram* of the process would look something like the graph that follows.

STRESS RESPONSE

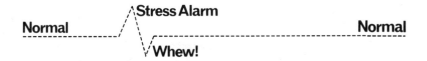

These large sawtooth jags of acute, short-term stress are part of regular living and are necessary for it. A certain amount of stress is needed to tune you for action and keep you on your toes, according to Dr. Hans Selye, the granddaddy of stress research who coined the term "stress" back in the 1940s.

*All diagrams originally prepared by Kenneth R. Pelletier, assistant clinical professor in the Department of Psychiatry at the University of California School of Medicine, San Francisco.

Normal Stress Can Spur You On

Acute stress can not only keep you on your toes—it can save your life. The surge of energy, concentration, and power that sudden stress brings can enable you to perform well beyond your normal capacities.

- A mother in Dorset, England, moved a 2000-pound car and saved her son who was pinned beneath—she weighed only 112 pounds.
- A weight lifter in Georgia was lying on his back, bench-pressing 250 pounds in his basement one Saturday when, exhausted, he dropped the weight onto his chest and could do nothing as it rolled onto his neck and began choking him. His sixty-pound, eleven-year-old daughter—the only one at home at the time— somehow managed to lift the 250-pound weight off her daddy enough so he could catch his breath and lift the weight the rest of the way off.
- A seventy-year-old man saw the car his twelve-year-old grand-daughter was riding in go over an embankment, managed to scramble down the slope after her and carry her up a hill so steep that a thirty-five-year-old relative who visited the accident site the following day said he could barely make it up alone and was convinced that it would be physically impossible to climb it carry-ing an unconscious, seventy-pound weight.

Stress can prod us to greater heights.

Bad Stress

But bad stress—chronic stress, distress day in and day out—will wear out the body and soul as surely as the drops from a leaking water tap can eat through a porcelain sink.

While the stress response is very useful if you have to fight off predators or escape a pursuer in a dark alley, for most of us it strikes when we are stuck behind a desk or sitting in a traffic jam. The ele-vated heartbeat simply leads to elevated blood pressure. Tensed mus-cles, when there is no pouncing or retreating to do, merely give you headaches and backaches and insomnia by the end of the day. The hormones that increase the tendency of the blood to clot—with no injury to attend to—just as likely lead to clots in coronary arteries. And the range of stress hormones, including epinephrine and norepinephrine, if not burned up in a burst of flight, build up in the blood to damage vessels and clog arteries, leading to heart disease—in some instances even sudden heart attacks.

The source of chronic stress can be found not so much in what we do each day but how we feel about it. Police officers, for example, complain that they experience more stress handling boring paperwork than they do while making arrests or responding to crimes in progress. They were trained to act, not sit and write, and that is what they feel competent doing. If we sense that we are not entirely in control of our lives, and every little move makes us anxious or dissatisfied and sends out a stress alarm, then we are never allowing ourselves the chance to say "Whew" and recuperate. It's the buildup of small but constant stress responses, not the occasional big ones, that inflicts the most bodily harm.

A diagram of chronic stress might look something like the graph below.

CHRONIC STRESS

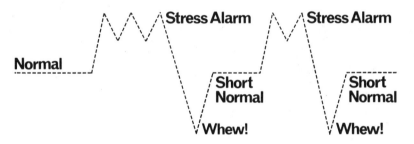

Whereas, a normal healthy life pattern might look something like this:

NORMAL STRESS

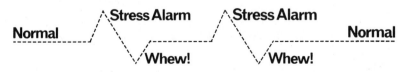

Stress lowers our immunity to infections and diseases. In a study of dental students taking exams, researchers at Harvard Medical School, Tufts University, and Beth Israel Hospital in Boston found that the students' levels of an important antibody (IGA, immunoglobulin-A) dropped. This antibody, circulating in saliva and other secretions, fights off viruses and bacteria that can lead to colds, respiratory diseases, bronchitis, even tooth decay.

Now most of us can bounce back from the temporary lowering of immunity under acute stress. The serious problems arise when we are under chronic stress—and lowered immunity leaves us constantly vulnerable.

Type A's Spell Distress

Type A personalities—the time-pressured, aggressive, angry people who have been found to be at higher risk for heart attacks and other stress-related diseases—put themselves under constant stress. As you'll see later, Type A persons feel that there is never enough time to do all they must, so they are always rushing, always under pressure to do more in less time, rarely enjoying their life as they live it, often feeling angry and hostile when others don't move fast enough. They never give themselves a chance to let up.

(See how you answered questions 9, 14, and 19 on the Stress Test as well as the questions listed in the sections on hostility and anger below, which are also characteristics of the Type A personality. The higher your score, the more Type A you are—and the higher your risk from stress-related diseases.)

Being Type A is not the price we have to pay for success. The truth is that being under constant low-level stress does not prod us on to greater heights—it wastes an enormous amount of energy and time. You can be far more productive, and probably a better manager of people as well, if you learn how to control those pressures instead of letting them control you. And the people who rise to the very top are more likely to have a larger share of calmer, more confident Type B characteristics than Type A traits.

Hostility and Anger Do You In

There are a number of emotions one can experience under stress, but anger and hostility seem to be the most self-destructive. Those who often feel a great deal of hostility (as measured by their responses to the Minnesota Multiphasic Personality Inventory, one of the oldest and most widely used tests in the psychological field) have a six times higher death rate from all causes—and a six times higher incidence of heart disease as well—than the average person. Men with higher hostility test scores have also been found to have significantly more blockage of coronary arteries than those with low scores.*

Are You Hostile?

See how you answered questions 1, 5, 12, and 22 on the Stress Test. Any total score of over 8 for just those questions means you would probably benefit by trying to reduce your hostile feelings. People who are very hostile are usually cynical, not very trusting, slightly paranoid in their human outlook. They are also likely to be angry.

Are You Angry?

See how you answered questions 3, 7, and 23 on the Stress Test. Any total score of over 6 for just those questions indicates you may be getting angry too often for your good health.

Anger is intimately linked with hostility—and likely just as self-destructive in triggering the dangerous effects of stress.

There has been much debate about whether to express anger or not, with the winds of pop psychology first blowing in the direction of letting it all hang out and then the revisionist wing coming out with the opposite notion that expressing your true feelings only makes everything worse. But as far as your health is concerned, the issue is not so much whether you should express anger as whether you should feel it so often in the first place. And, for your health, the emerging consensus is that the less you feel, the better. It's no good feeling it and then not mentioning it and pretending you didn't. Nor is it helpful to feel anger and then keep the fires burning as you explain in exquisite detail why you were and still are seething.

As long as you are angry, you are triggering the body's stress response and you are suffering from the wear and tear that the stress hormones bring. Now that doesn't mean you should never get angry—

---

*Redford Williams, a professor of psychiatry and associate professor of internal medicine at Duke University, conducted these studies on hostility, which he and others are continuing to explore.

no extreme is healthy. But you have to choose which circumstances are worth it, instead of letting petty problems keep you under chronic stress.

It is normal to feel anger and hostility sometimes. And it is hard to change those reflexes. But recognizing the adverse health consequences of such reactions and realizing that they are rarely productive can help you cut your anger short.

At least you should know that if anger puts you at risk, you would be well advised to compensate by cutting back on some other health risk—smoke less or drink less or exercise more.

Grief

Grieving for someone you loved, while natural, also puts you under stress—and lowers your immunity to disease. Widows and widowers have much higher rates of sickness and death than others of the same age. An Australian study has shown that the intense grieving during the eight weeks following the death of their spouses lowered the immune responses of widows and widowers and left them more vulnerable to infection and cancer. A New York study* found suppressed lymphocyte activity (a critical part of the immune system) in men whose wives had died of breast cancer in the last six weeks.

That does not mean that the 700,000 people over age fifty who lose spouses every year in the United States should sit back and wait for death or disease to take them, too. For the bereaved as well as for people with Type A character traits, or people who know they feel largely out of control and dissatisfied with their lives, the point here is to face that you are at heightened risk—and then make changes to lower that risk.

There are many things you can do. No one can bring back a spouse or change one's parents, if they, too, were Type A and trained you well (as explained in chapter 13, Type A behavior is more a learned pattern of behavior than an inherited one). But we can recognize, as John Milton said, "The mind is its own place and in itself can make a heaven of hell, a hell of heaven." We can control our attitudes about how we live and who's in charge. Often it takes only a few small steps to set our health patterns right.

---

*The research was conducted by Steven Schleifer and colleagues at Mount Sinai School of Medicine in New York City.

Good Stress to the Rescue

The best revenge is living well—and the best counter for distress is the experience of positive emotions.

Successfully rising to the challenge—even if one initially felt acute stress at the challenge—and afterward feeling that glow of confidence and a sense of control over one's destiny seem to go a long way toward counteracting the ill effects of stress—it may even help cure disease.

Success Is Counted Sweetest . . .

High-powered, successful men and women may work hard and long, but they are not doing themselves in by it—if they enjoy their success. Success is a powerful defuser of stress. In 1974, the Metropolitan Life Insurance Company examined 1078 men who held one of the three top executive positions in Fortune 500 companies and found that their mortality rate was 37 percent lower than that of other white males of a comparable age.

The explanation may reside in a study of 259 executives at Illinois Bell conducted by a psychologist at the University of Chicago. She found that certain people seemed to be particularly able to handle stress, staying healthy no matter how intense their job pressures or how ominous their family medical history. And what enabled them to cope seemed to be common attitudes: they all felt a sense of purpose, viewed change as a challenge and not a threat, and believed they were in control of their lives.

Executive women—presumably under a great deal of stress to make it in the corporate world—must feel some of this sense of control. Recent studies show no sign that their push into the upper ranks is causing their health to suffer. Metropolitan Life's 1979 study of 2352 women listed in *Who's Who* showed their annual death rate to be 29 percent lower than that of their contemporaries.

It is simply a myth that if you work like a man you'll die like a man. Even with an unprecedented number of women in the work force today, mortality rates for coronary heart disease are declining faster for women than men. Indeed, the highest rates of heart disease are among secretaries and saleswomen, not the hotshot executives—again, these are the women with little job security, status or control.

Symphony conductors, for example, undergo great physical exertion: traveling, meeting deadlines, dealing with temperamental musicians in the orchestra. But they are also proud of their achievements, they are respected by everyone in the music world, they are applauded by audiences. And the result is that they live much longer, healthier lives than the average person.

Happiness, A Stable Love Life, Can Outweigh Bad Habits

Being happily married or attached, and developing good friendships, for example, can even overcome some of the ill effects of bad physical habits, such as overeating.

Residents of Roseto, Pennsylvania, a largely Italian community sixty miles outside of New York City, regularly eat a diet higher in fats and calories than people in surrounding communities—but they have no higher blood cholesterol levels and one-third as many heart attacks. Why? Perhaps because these 1630 people (studied by cardiologist Dr. Stewart Wolf in the 1960s) live in a cohesive, mutually supportive community with strong family ties. There is no crime or poverty. And most of the men over twenty-five are married. (Men and women who are married show much lower incidences of disease and premature death than single or divorced individuals.)

Love, friendships, and social support defuse stress—even among animals. Experiments have shown that mice injected with cancer cells and then isolated from other mice will develop tumors more rapidly than those who are likewise injected but remain with their cage mates.

Laughter as Medicine—Good Stress May Reverse Damage

The idea that laughter and positive emotions are good for us has been floating around for centuries. It has a commonsense appeal. We all know the glorious drained, relaxed feeling that follows a good roar, and intuitively appreciate that anxiety cannot possibly exist when you feel so limp-muscled and serene. Norman Cousins, the outspoken proponent of laughter as good medicine, believes it actually helped save his life when he became very ill. Mark Twain, too, understood:

". . . the old man laughed loud and joyously, shook up the details of his anatomy from head to foot, and ended by saying that such a laugh was money in a man's pocket, because it cut down the doctor's bills like everything." *(Tom Sawyer)*

Today, such notions about the good effects of laughter and other positive emotions are being elevated above folk wisdom and scientifically investigated. At first glance, laughter seems to trigger physical reactions that are much like the stress response. Hard laughter puts the body through a good physical workout—Norman Cousins calls it "internal jogging." The oxygen supply to the brain increases, heartbeat speeds up, pupils dilate, muscles tense, and so on.

But something different may be going on at the biochemical level. Endorphins, the body's natural painkillers, are being released. Endorphins are 20 to 100 times as powerful as morphine and do more than relieve pain—they play a role in memory and learning, sexual activity, control of body temperature, and the regulation of other hormones. And what scientists are currently exploring is the possibility that more of these hormones and others may be secreted under good stress than under normal or bad stress, and that they may actually reverse some of the damage of the distress reaction.

New, ultrasensitive measuring equipment is starting to show differences in skin temperature and heart rate between those experiencing sadness and happiness, as well as a range of other emotions, though each can provoke something similar to the stress response, and each can even move you to tears. The chemicals released in the stress response seem to vary subtly depending upon whether you feel happy or sad, nervous but basically confident that you can cope, or nervous but fearful that you can't. Finally the old notion that has dominated the stress field—the notion that stress involves the same response to change regardless of whether the change is a happy or sad event—is being challenged.

We know that bad (chronic) stress can lower the effectiveness of our immune responses, making us more vulnerable to everything from colds and flu to cancer. There is evidence (according to Dr. Paul Rosch, cardiologist and president of the American Stress Institute in Yonkers, New York, among others) that the cell walls of lymphocytes—which lead our immune systems in the fight against viruses and cancer—have receptor sites for ACTH (one of the prime stress hormones), endorphins, metenkephalin, and other brain hormones. This implies that the brain can talk directly to the immune system and that the immune system talks back. If we can learn how to get in on this conversation—just as humans have learned to influence such bodily processes as pulse rate and heartbeat and skin temperature which a decade ago few thought we could do voluntarily—then we may be able to stimulate our immune system when we are ill. Or we may be able to calm it down from overreacting, as it does in autoimmune diseases such as arthritis, allergies, lupus, and after artificial organ transplants or skin grafts.

In short, just as we know bad stress can make us ill, there is a strong possibility that good stress may be just as potent in making us well.

And there are many easy steps we can take to convert our bad stress to good—and to stop killing ourselves.

How to Convert Bad Stress to Good

That's exactly what chapters 12 and 13 explain. You will find out:

1. The early-warning signs of stress. Bad stress begins long before most of us realize it. Look for: cold hands, sweaty palms, shortness of breath, unexplained moodiness, burping, indigestion, becoming accident-prone, insomnia.
2. How to change your Type A ways.
3. How to wait in line without stress.
4. How to master the Ten-Second Stress Fix and other relaxation techniques.
5. How to talk to yourself to encourage success and defuse stress.
6. How daydreaming and visualization can help you modify behavior.
7. Suggestions for an Antistress Diet and Antistress Exercises.

6
Heart Disease

ALEXANDER IS A TYPICAL healthy little boy. He loves to chase bubbles. He says he can "run like the wind." And though he doesn't feel a thing and may show no symptoms for decades to come, at this moment—as he blows out the three candles on his birthday cake and his mother passes out the ice cream—fat is beginning to clog the blood vessels that keep him alive.

By age three, almost all American children have streaks of fat building up in their aortas, the main artery that feeds the body with its lifeblood, a startling piece of medical information stumbled upon accidentally in the course of post-mortem studies of children who died accidentally.

By age eleven, over half of all schoolchildren have serious—though usually silent—signs of cardiovascular dangers building : In a survey * of 2500 eleven- to fourteen-year-olds, close to one in five had high cholesterol and were at least 20 percent overweight; 25 percent smoked regularly, and 5 percent had high blood pressure.

By twenty-two, even those as healthy and fit as young soldiers have been found (when autopsied) to have at least one of three main coronary arteries 25 percent blocked with fat and cholesterol.

The vast majority of Americans have some accumulation of fatty deposits that harden and clog the arteries—atherosclerosis—long before there are any warning signs. It can happen anywhere in the body: if the blockage is in the arteries that supply blood and nourishment to the heart, it can cause a heart attack; if it's along the path to the brain, it can cause a stroke; if to the legs, it interferes with walking; if to the genitals, it upsets sexual performance . . . and so on.

---

* These children were participating in the American Health Foundation's nationwide "Know Your Body" program.

It is not surprising, then, that cardiovascular diseases—all the ailments of the heart and blood vessels that we commonly lump under "heart problems," but which, in addition to heart attacks include strokes, atherosclerosis, and hypertension—are the number one killers today.

But what might surprise many is that this need not be so. Heart disease, especially before age fifty or sixty, is not a necessary part of the human condition.

Heart Disease Can Be Prevented

We can prevent most heart attacks. This statement may not sound revolutionary today but it reveals a complete turnaround in approach from what doctors practicing today were taught as recently as two decades ago. Medical students in the 1960s, according to one of them who went on to serve as the head of the preventive cardiology branch of the National Heart, Lung, and Blood Institute in Washington, D.C., were taught that there was little anyone could do for those whose genes made them susceptible to heart disease. Smoking had not yet been conclusively linked to heart disease.

Now the medical profession and all of us know better.

Our Way of Life Shapes Our Way of Death

The evidence seems stronger with each new study that the changes in life-style in the twentieth century are what has made heart disease the leading killer. At the turn of the century, heart disease was a rarity. Until the 1920s, a doctor could spend an entire career in one community and see perhaps one or two patients suffering heart attacks.

Heart disease was rare not because people didn't live long enough to wear out this hardworking organ, but because they lived differently. Forty percent of Americans lived on small farms, plowing, planting, milking from sunup to sundown. (Less than 4 percent of the population today are farmers.) And those not on farms routinely walked miles daily into town for school, shopping, socializing. Few smoked, and they ate largely what they and their neighbors grew and preserved. Only the well-to-do could afford large helpings of meat and refined white sugar and flour.

By the 1940s, industrialization changed Americans' lives further, concentrating them in the cities. The automobile reduced physical activity. The smoking habit spread as only fire can, and modern food processing changed diets—sometimes for the better, but not often. Heart disease soared. And it didn't decrease at all (despite the many advances made in medical technology) until after the 1964 surgeon general's report publicized the link between cigarette smoking and heart disease and prompted great numbers of people to kick the habit.

Today, heart disease is continuing to decline, precisely because we are changing our behavior and daily habits for the better. People are exercising more, eating less butter and fewer eggs, shunning cigarettes. At least some people are—but not enough.

Heart disease still kills three times as many people as cancer. It afflicts over 40 million Americans. Well over a million people die every year from heart-related problems. These disorders don't just kill, they rank first in disabling people, limiting their activity, causing them to lose workdays and generally making life more miserable than it need be.

The Broken-Hearted

- Heart attacks: 1,250,000 Americans a year have heart attacks; 650,000 die of heart disease—and over one-third of those die well before their time should really be up: under age 65.
- Strokes: More than 183,000 die of stroke, and those who survive are often severely handicapped.
- Hypertension: Some 60 million suffer elevated blood pressure (over 140/90) and 35 million have high blood pressure (over 160/95), which can increase the risk for both of the above diseases and more.

The Heart—a Hardworking Organ

This amazing muscle, about the size of your fist, beats 100,000 times a day, pumping about 4000 gallons of blood through 60,000 miles of blood vessels throughout the body. Every thirteen seconds the heart propels a fresh supply of blood and oxygen to every cell in the body—and it rarely misfires or gets tired. If all else went smoothly in our bodies, the heart itself could probably go on pumping for well over a hundred years. Most of the problems we label heart disease do not stem from the functioning of the heart so much as the blood vessels leading to or from the heart.

What Is a Heart Attack?

A heart attack (also called a myocardial infarction or a coronary thrombosis) occurs when the blood supply to some portion of the heart is cut. This can happen in a number of ways. Most commonly, the arteries feeding the heart become blocked by a buildup of cholesterol and plaque (a condition called atherosclerosis) which prevents blood from reaching the heart. Those same arteries, whether clogged or clear, can also go into spasm, choking off the heart's lifeblood. The ventricles (pumping chambers) of the heart can also go into spasm (called fibrillation) and cause a heart attack.

Atherosclerosis (hardening of the arteries), however, seems to be the main culprit in heart disease and heart attacks. The term derives from the Greek word *athera* meaning "gruel," which describes the sticky yellow cholesterol that collects in atherosclerotic arteries.

These cholesterol globs combine with other substances to form plaque that begins building silently in arteries from birth. The more fat and cholesterol in our diets, the faster and heavier the buildup. A middle-aged person may have a coronary artery more than 50 percent blocked (these arteries are only about one-eighth of an inch in diameter to begin with) without feeling any symptoms. By the time we feel the pain of angina pectoris—the squeezing, constricting feeling in the chest, arm, or shoulder that comes when the heart isn't getting all the blood and oxygen it needs—the arteries are usually 80 to 90 percent blocked.

Some people never experience angina or notice any other warning signs. For half the people, the first heart attack is the last. Even for those who survive, there is no way to reverse the heart attack's damage—dead muscle tissue, or dead brain cells in the case of a stroke. A mild heart attack kills 20 percent of the heart muscle, a severe one can destroy as much as 70 percent.

Recovery is possible. But prevention—by making small adjustments in our daily habits, that will be detailed later, to keep the blood in our vessels flowing freely—is not only safer but also more effective than current mopping-up procedures for those with heart disease.

Diet and exercise, smoking and drinking, personality, all play a part in the buildup of plaque (fatty clumps in the arteries) and hypertension. And emotional stress—not sudden shocks so much as the chronic feeling of being under stress—is coming to be recognized as a significant contributor to our risks. Under stress, the body releases epinephrine (which used to be called adrenaline) and norepinephrine. These chemicals constrict blood vessels, increase heart and blood-pressure rates, damage artery linings, making them more susceptible to the buildup of plaque, stimulate blood clotting which can obstruct the flow of blood, and perhaps even trigger ventricular spasm. In short, the stress chemicals can lead to both slow and sudden death.

What Is a Stroke?

When bleeding or a blood clot blocks the supply of oxygen to the brain, a stroke results. The clot can lodge in arteries damaged by atherosclerosis (cerebral thrombosis) or it can wander in the bloodstream and then settle in an artery leading to the brain (cerebral embolism). Or a defective artery in the brain (defective usually from the wear and tear of high blood pressure or atherosclerosis) can burst, depriving the brain of its necessary blood supply (cerebral hemorrhage).

Over 500,000 people suffer strokes each year; more than 170,000 die, and many survivors never fully recover.

The body may or may not reveal two early-warning signs: hypertension is the first signal of possible trouble ahead. The second is an incident that mimics an actual stroke but does not do permanent damage. The experience usually lasts about twenty minutes, making the victim see double, slur speech, feel numb or paralyzed in an arm or leg or in the face. But unlike the symptoms of a genuine stroke, this effect is short-lived. Many people dismiss such an episode, but it is always a mistake to ignore messages the body tries to send out.

Stroke is the third leading cause of death—but frightening as these mortality statistics may be, they don't even paint the full picture. Most stroke victims survive—but many spend their remaining years seriously crippled.

What Is Hypertension?

This disorder, also known as high blood pressure, is often called the silent killer because it has no obvious bodily symptoms. People with high blood pressure have five times the incidence of heart failure as those with normal pressure, seven times as many strokes.

In people with high blood pressure, the arteries become narrow, forcing the heart to pump harder than normal to keep the blood flowing throughout the body. Eventually the heart muscle becomes larger as a result of working overtime, and its needs for oxygen increase. When those needs cannot be met, the heart's gasp for oxygen turns into a heart attack.

With the heart pumping hard, pressure against the blood vessel walls increases, possibly weakening and damaging those walls. Damaged walls seem to attract fatty plaque; the buildup of plaque further narrows the vessel walls and pushes blood pressure up even higher. If this cycle continues without interruption, the weakened blood vessels may eventually burst, producing either a heart attack or a stroke.

Hormones, other chemicals, and nerve cells constantly change the width of the arteries to adapt to life's little curves—heat, cold, pregnancy, and so on. (The "rosy glow of pregnancy," for example, probably has less to do with a woman's anticipating the joys of motherhood than it does with her hormones widening blood vessels—many located near the surface of the "rosy" skin—to accommodate the 50 percent increase in blood flow that pregnancy brings. Sentimentality dealt another blow.)

But most important, the width of the arteries also depends upon how much fatty plaque—resulting from high-fat diets, chronic stress, insufficient exercise, smoking, and so on—builds up to clog those passageways. Reducing blockage can reduce blood pressure.

Some 35 million Americans have high blood pressure, which, according to the World Health Organization, means blood pressure over 160/95. Another 25 million Americans have elevated blood pressure, over 140/90, which puts them at increased risk of illness and death. And because the only ways to uncover high blood pressure in the early stages is to take a blood-pressure reading, many more people have the disorder without knowing it.

What Do the Blood-Pressure Numbers Mean?

Blood pressure is measured in millimeters of mercury (mmHg) and really must be measured several times at different points in the day to get an accurate reading.

The higher number is a measure of the force with which the heart pushes blood out to the body as it contracts, called the systolic blood pressure. The lower number represents the resistance of the blood vessels to the flow of blood as the heart relaxes between beats, called the diastolic pressure. For example, 120/80 is considered normal; if yours is above that, you should check with a doctor on steps to take.

Most Americans find that their systolic blood pressure rises with age until ages forty-five to fifty, then it begins to drop again. But rising blood pressure is not an inevitable accompaniment to aging—rural populations have been found to maintain constant blood pressure all their lives.

Tips On Getting Accurate BP Readings

- Do not talk while taking your blood pressure or for several minutes beforehand—your blood pressure rises 10 to 50 percent above normal about half a minute after you start talking.
- Get a reading at the hands of both a doctor and a nurse. Blood pressure rises most steeply when a person perceives that the person he or she is talking to is of higher status, according to studies by Dr. James Lynch at the University of Maryland School of Medicine.

Are You at Risk?

What are the causes of cardiovascular disease? Inherited susceptibility plays a part, but even more important seem to be our habits—what we eat, how we move, whether we smoke, and how we typically react to the ordinary stresses of life—in short, what we do with ourselves and to ourselves day in and day out.

Take this test and see if you're at risk.

HEART TEST

1. If you are male   *Add 2.*
   If you are female   *Add 0.*
2. You are over 55   *Add 2.*
   You are over 40   *Add 1.*
   You are under 40   *Add 0.*
3. If you smoke:
   Two packs or more a day   *Add 20.*
   One to 2 packs a day   *Add 12.*
   More than 5 cigars a day or inhale on a pipe regularly
   Add 12.

Nothing now, but quit smoking less than a year ago   *Add 10.*
Less than 1 pack   *Add 6.*
Less than 6 cigars, or an occasional pipe   *Add 6.*
Nothing, but quit smoking less than 10 years ago   *Add 3.*
Nothing, but quit over 10 years ago or never smoked   *Add 0.*

4. You have high blood pressure (over 160/100)   *Add 20.*
   You have elevated blood pressure (over 140/90)   *Add 10.*
   Your blood pressure is normal (under 140/90)   *Add 0.*

5. You are more than 20 percent overweight (that's 30 pounds if you should weigh 150, or 22 pounds if you should weigh 110)   *Add 10.*
   You are more than 10 percent overweight   *Add 5.*
   You are within 10 pounds of your ideal weight   *Add 0.*

6. If you are under constant tension, feeling rushed, pressured, easily irritated throughout the day   *Add 10.*
   If you are under deadline pressure, but usually manage to do your work with only occasional flare-ups or occasionally feeling great tension   *Add 5.*
   If you usually feel relaxed and calm and unhurried   *Add 0.*

7. (Pick whichever comes closest to your diet habits; "dessert" here means something along the lines of cake/cookies/ice cream.)
   You eat red meat at least once daily, use butter, rarely margarine, whole milk and cheese, eggs often, and desserts several times a week   *Add 20.*
   You eat red meat less than 5 times a week, use margarine more often than butter, and eat modest amounts of cheese and eggs, and dessert less than three times a week   *Add 10.*
   You eat red meat less than three times a week (eating fish and poultry or vegetables instead), margarine and that only modestly, skim-milk cheeses, fewer than three eggs a week, and desserts less than once a week   *Add 0.*

8. If your cholesterol count is higher than 280   *Add 20.*
   If it is over 220 but under 280   *Add 10.*
   (This is the range the average American falls into.)
   If it is below 220   *Add 0.*

9. If you exercise vigorously for 30 minutes at least 3 times a week   *Add 0.*
   If you exercise vigorously for 30 minutes twice a week   *Add 5.*
   If you exercise vigorously less than once a week   *Add 10.*

10. You'd describe yourself as an ambitious, hard-driving person, with a fiery temper, who feels as if you're wasting time if not

working on at least two things at once, at work and at play
Add 10.

You'd describe yourself as a hard-driving person who gets irritated easily under pressure, but who can relax away from the office   *Add 5.*

You are an even-tempered person who enjoys work but enjoys playing as well, who can function under competition but prefers a more relaxed atmosphere   *Add 0.*

11. You have diabetes, take insulin, and are under 40   *Add 20.*
    You have diabetes, use some drug treatment, and are over 40   *Add 10.*
    Your diabetes began after age 55 and is under control with diet   *Add 5.*

12. Your mother or father had a heart attack or stroke before age 60   *Add 22.*
    Your mother or father had heart disease before 60 but no heart attacks or strokes   *Add 18.*
    Your mother or father had a heart attack or stroke after age 60   *Add 12.*

13. You have had a heart attack, a blocked blood vessel, or a stroke before age 50   *Add 40.*
    You have had a heart attack, a blocked blood vessel, or a stroke after age 50   *Add 20.*

14. If you are married   *Add 0.*
    If you are separated, divorced, or widowed   *Add 10.*

15. You are not happy about the work you do, and you are troubled about how things are going in your personal life as well   *Add 10.*
    You are not happy about your work but you have at least one person you love, and who helps you through tough times   *Add 5.*
    Most of the time you are happy about the work you do and about your homelife as well   *Add 0.*

Test Score

High risk—Over 95.
Medium risk—45–95.
Low risk—Below 45.

Risk Factors for Heart Disease Beyond Your Control

There are certain hereditary risk factors you can't change. But you ought to know about them in order to gain a realistic picture of your own risks—and to motivate you even more strongly to change those factors you can control.

Family history certainly plays a part in heart disease. If you have parents or aunts and uncles who had heart attacks before age sixty, then you are considered at higher risk than normal.

Hypertension in parents puts children at twice the normal risk of developing hypertension. However, many hypertension specialists suspect this results not so much from a genetic inheritance as an environmental one—eating patterns, exercise habits, ways of coping with stress that parents teach their children. Families in which the father is hypertensive have been shown in studies not to discuss conflicts when they arise. The parents, and their children who follow their example, simply stew and let their blood pressure go haywire.

Firstborn children also have been found to be at higher risk for developing hypertension later in life. Again, this factor may have something to do with the more intense pressure to achieve that firstborns often feel.

Gender counts, too—men have about twice as great a risk of heart disease as women. But that does not mean women are immune. Women are about ten years behind men—so a forty-year-old woman faces about as much heart-disease risk as a thirty-year-old man. After age sixty, the gap between men and women starts to close.

However, at any age, if women smoke or display any other serious risk factors, the gender gap evaporates.

Race is a factor as well—black men in American have three times the incidence of hypertension that white men have, and black women have twice the incidence of white women. Black people's rate of heart attacks and strokes is also higher than whites. Again, debate continues on this risk factor as to whether the source of the problem is in the genes or in something more subjective such as the socioeconomic circumstances of the majority of blacks in America and the associated pressures and frustrations those circumstances bring.

Asians in the United States have a lower rate of heart attacks than whites but a higher rate than Asians living in China and Japan.

Age is never irrelevant—the older you get, the higher your risk. And elevated blood pressure (which usually accompanies getting older) increases the risk of heart attack and stroke, even before it reaches the levels classified as "high."

Height may also prove to be a factor, though findings here are quite tentative. A British study found that coronary mortality was 54 percent greater in men who were under 5 feet 6 inches than those over 6 feet. It may have something to do with a deficiency in the growth hormone (HGH) or it may be that shorter men develop unusually aggressive, Type A personalities to compensate for their size.

But recognizing these seemingly immutable factors—no matter how many you share—should only give you more incentive to change the things you can.

I. Type A Personality

RISK FACTORS YOU CAN CONTROL

"Regardless of fatty foods eaten, cigarettes smoked, or lack of exercise, coronary heart disease almost never occurs before age 70 in the absence of Type A behavior," wrote Drs. Meyer Friedman and Ray Rosenman back in 1974 when they first identified this personality trait that makes one highly vulnerable to heart disease. And the evidence in the decade since seems to support their assertion that Type A's have two to three times the chances of developing heart disease as calmer, less time-pressured Type Bs.

The Type A personality belongs to people aggressively involved in a chronic struggle to achieve more and more in less and less time. They schedule more into a day than can possibly be done and always feel rushed as a result; they often use sharp, explosive speech patterns and hand gestures (pounding their fists, pointing); and they become angry or hostile readily though the casual observer may not notice this trait in them and they may be the last to know themselves.

Type A behavior may be the single crucial factor in coronary disease between the ages of thirty and forty-five, when about one-third of all heart attacks strike.

Type A women are at risk, too, not just the men. At any age, women with Type A personalities have about twice the risk of heart disease as women with calmer, Type B personalities, according to statistics gathered by a behavioral epidemiologist at the National Heart, Lung, and Blood Institute. And research, for the first time, has also demonstrated the link between Type A personality and stroke. Type A women have been found to be at higher risk for stroke than

Type B women and than Type B men. (Men and women, on average, usually have about the same incidence of stroke.)

The Type A personality may be hazardous to your health—largely because it has been widely misunderstood. It is called a "personality," and it has been found to run in families—but it is by no means a genetic trait. The uptight, time-pressured Type A personality is, as the cardiologists who coined the term insist, a cluster of behaviors that are far more learned from parents, teachers, and observing others than inherited. By example, Type A fathers and mothers teach their children to respond to the stresses of life with Type A behavior. And Western culture, which rewards workaholics who perform rapidly and aggressively, reinforces Type A tendencies in us all.

But if you have become a Type A, you do not have to stay that way forever. Type A personality traits are not set in stone. You can modify your behavior—and even small changes may be the most critical steps in protecting against heart disease.

WHY TYPE A BEHAVIOR CAUSES DAMAGE

The exact biochemical mechanisms that put Type As at risk have not been definitively traced yet. But there are clues.

Type A's may have blood pressure that is as low when resting as Type Bs. Recent research reveals that the irregularities arise only when they are involved in a task that they regard as stressful. Then the Type A secretes unusually high levels of epinephrine and nor-epinephrine; these hormones—released under stress—raise blood pressure, damage the lining of arteries, and can even trigger sudden heart attacks.

The problem is that Type A's react as if they are under stress nearly all the time. When facing even the smallest event, they respond with an excessive outpouring of stress hormones. And when the body experiences this hormonal onslaught day in and day out, year after year, the heart and blood vessels eventually have to pay the price.

The tricky element here is that Type A's may not display high blood pressure or any other irregularities under calm conditions—just under stress. This may help explain why someone at serious risk can go to a doctor's office, get a clean bill of health, and then have a heart attack on the way out.

Usually, however, Type A's and others at risk do get any number of warning signals from their systems—if they only knew what to look for, and if they only paid attention. Type A behavior patterns in themselves constitute a very large and very serious set of warning signals.

Remember again, Type A traits are not immutable. They are behavior, much like good or bad manners, that you have learned and acquired; and while you may not be able to "unlearn" them completely, you can most definitely modify your Type A tendencies—and save your life. In a study of people who had already suffered heart attacks, preliminary findings are that their chances of suffering second ones go down 50 percent if they change *some* of their Type A traits.

Whether you are Type A or not, there are a number of other important risk factors you can begin to control—and reduce—right now.

II. Diet

Diet counts—what you eat, and how much of it as well. Cutting blood cholesterol levels 10 percent can cut heart disease risks by 30 percent. If everyone simply weighed within the normal range for his or her height and age, there would be 24 percent less heart disease and 35 percent less congestive heart failure and stroke.

Once you decide which foods you want to eat or avoid, you can turn to chapter 15 on diet for additional advice on palatable and painless food substitutions.

Now for the specifics.

CHOLESTEROL AND FATS

In a study of heart-disease mortality in seven countries, the highest death rates among the middle-aged prevailed in eastern Finland and the United States, where the saturated fat and cholesterol in the diet were the highest. The lowest recorded death rates were in the Greek islands of Corfu and Crete, Dalmatia in Yugoslavia, and Japan—all regions where the diets are low in fat.

Fat consumption in the United States rose 25 percent from the turn of the century to the 1970s. Now it is going down. So is heart disease. We are still eating a higher percentage of fat in our diets than we should, but many are taking the first step—reducing fats, especially saturated fats.

Animal fats are the major source of cholesterol, consisting largely of saturated fatty acids that are solid at room temperature. Vegetable oils, while containing the same number of calories, are primarily made up of polyunsaturated fatty acids (coconut and palm oil are the saturated exceptions) and contain little or no cholesterol. Polyunsaturates seem to lower cholesterol levels in the blood, while saturates raise it and thereby endanger the heart.

Cholesterol has become a dirty word. But its bad reputation as a substance that will clog up our arteries and lead to heart disease is only partially deserved. Cholesterol has good and bad points.

We can't do without some of it. Cholesterol forms vitamin D in the skin, which ultimately helps synthesize a number of hormones, including sex hormones and bile acids needed for digestion. That's why the body doesn't wait around for its supply to come from the food we eat; it produces about 200 milligrams of this waxy substance on its own every day.

But precisely because the body produces a great deal of cholesterol, we don't need to consume very much in our diets before we begin to suffer from cholesterol overload.

How does fat get from your mouth to the bloodstream?

As fatty foods are eaten and broken down, some of the fat is used for energy and cell growth. Some, sad to say, is stored. The rest is carried into the bloodstream. At first, the fat appears as streaks in the arteries; later it builds up into plaques (fatty clumps), which lean against the artery walls like a schoolyard bully, getting larger and tougher with each fatty meal and increasingly obstructing the flow of blood vital to the heart.

Once cholesterol enters the bloodstream, it hooks up with special proteins that lead it around in its new form as either high-density lipoprotein (HDL) or low-density lipoprotein (LDL). HDL reduces cholesterol levels in the blood by leading the cholesterol out of the body; LDL causes trouble by allowing the cholesterol to loiter in the vessels and clog up the free flow of blood.

For men, keeping blood vessels clear by cutting back on fats and cholesterol could extend sex life as well. The testicles are especially susceptible to atherosclerosis. The arteries lying over the outer shell of the testicle enter the body at a sharp angle—and anywhere there are angles, fatty deposits can develop. When fatty deposits reduce blood supplies, the deprived cells and organs don't work up to par.

HOW DO YOU LOWER CHOLESTEROL LEVELS IN THE BLOOD?

If you were born female, you have a built-in advantage. Women's hormones give them a higher proportion of HDL to LDL, which may partially account for their much lower incidence of heart disease.

If you've already missed that chance, then you'll have to lower cholesterol levels through diet and exercise.

The rule of thumb here is to eat less of all fats, not just saturated animal fats but polyunsaturated fats as well. And the easiest way to do this is to cut back on red meat—which is quite high in fat—and get your protein instead from chicken, fish, and a mixture of grains and vegetables that can supply complete proteins. Also, quit worrying about loading up on proteins—most Americans get plenty. What we need more of are fruits and vegetables, which contain large amounts of vitamins and minerals but few calories.

Yogurt seems to help lower cholesterol levels, even though it is made from milk and thus contains saturated fats.

Eggs and shellfish—recently under attack for being high in cholesterol—have gotten a nastier reputation than they deserve. While eggs are very high in cholesterol, they are also a good, cheap, low-calorie source of protein. And the white, which has about as much protein as the yolk, has no cholesterol or fat at all.

Shellfish, too, are lower in calories and fat than equivalent portions of meat. And while it is true that shrimp is fairly high in cholesterol, lobster is no higher than chicken.

Furthermore, the amount of cholesterol one consumes does not affect blood levels of cholesterol as significantly as the amount of fat.

FAT AND HYPERTENSION

Low-fat diets, with less saturated than polyunsaturated fats, can reduce blood pressure. But blood pressure stays down only as long as you stay on the diet.

FAT'S WORSE THAN SMOKING

Eating a fatty diet seems to be worse than smoking. The Japanese, who smoke heavily, still have the lowest incidence of heart disease among the developed nations. The reason may be that they have a very low-fat diet—10 percent of their calories come from fat as compared to 40 percent for the average American. Average cholesterol levels among Japanese are 150 milligrams per deciliter as compared to 220 plus for Americans.

The Japanese immunity to heart disease is not genetic—they lose it when they move to countries like America and begin eating like the Americans—diets high in fat and cholesterol.

The Japanese diet is still not the ideal—they, too, have a lot to learn. They eat large amounts of salt and consequently also have a high incidence of hypertension and stroke.

ATHEROSCLEROSIS AND VITAMIN B-6

Another theory about the buildup of fats in blood vessels points the accusatory finger away from cholesterol and at diets too low in B-6, which is thought to help clear out homocysteine, a chemical in the blood that encourages atherosclerosis. Thus, according to this theory, one should consume foods that have a high ratio of vitamin B-6 to methionine, the dietary source of homocysteine: these include bananas, avocados, oranges, lettuce, tomatoes, potatoes, spinach, carrots.

Anywhere from 50 to 90 percent of B-6 is lost in cooking; much is also lost in milling wheat to make white flour; canned foods have about two-thirds less B-6 than their fresh, uncooked counterparts. It isn't hard to see how a normal American diet might easily be low in B-6.

Women on the pill, and women who are menstruating or pregnant may be especially low in B-6. Aside from the buildup of cholesterol, this deficiency can cause cramps. For most people, consuming from 5 to 50 milligrams a day of B-6 should be ample. Taking higher-dose supplements may not do great harm, as the body excretes what it cannot use, but it can be a waste of money.

OVERWEIGHT

The more overweight you are, the greater your risk for hypertension and heart disease. People who are 20 percent overweight have been found to have eight times higher risk of developing hypertension than those 10 percent overweight. For men between the ages of thirty-five and fifty-five, a 10 percent weight reduction can bring about a 20 percent reduction in the incidence of coronary disease.

SALT

Some researchers have gone so far as to say that if salt were eliminated from the diet, hypertension would practically disappear. For those who already show signs of hypertension or are at high risk, cutting down on salt unquestionably lowers risks.

But the latest evidence goes even further, suggesting that healthy people—even newborns with no apparent problems—who eat a low-salt diet (the newborns were given a low-salt formula; yes, even formula has salt added) can lower their blood pressure.

If you're interested in some salt substitutes that keep food flavorful, turn to chapter 15.

ALCOHOL

Alcohol raises blood pressure. Perhaps 10 percent of hypertension may result from excessive alcohol consumption.

On the other hand, a glass or two of wine a day may help to lower the LDL, or "bad" cholesterol levels in the blood.

The debate over alcohol and the heart continues. There have been other widely publicized studies suggesting that drinking two or three drinks a day can ward off coronary heart disease—one Hawaiian study projected by as much as five to ten years. Appealing though many of us may find those reports, there are even more studies that contradict them. Besides, alcohol can increase cancer risk, damage the heart muscle and the liver, and increase the risk of automobile and other accidents. Moderation, once again, is the safest path.

CAFFEINE

Caffeine temporarily raises blood pressure. And it may also increase cholesterol levels in the blood. Though studies have leaned both ways on the coffee-cholesterol link, one recent investigation found that drinking four cups of coffee can raise cholesterol 5 percent; drinking five to eight cups can raise it 9 percent; and drinking nine or more cups produces a 12 percent jump in cholesterol.

Consuming large amounts of caffeine also seems to increase the urge to drink alcohol—though no one can say exactly why this seems to be the case. It may be that the caffeine makes you feel so nervous and jumpy by the end of the day that you want a drink to calm down. While the data are more speculative than scientific, if you find that you want to cut back on alcohol in the evening, you might first cut back on caffeine during the day.

CALCIUM

Calcium helps lower blood pressure, according to a study by the Johns Hopkins School of Medicine and investigators from the Institute of Nutrition of Central America and Panama. One-gram calcium supplements taken daily in this study lowered blood pressure in healthy young adults.

Unfortunately, in an effort to cut out fatty foods, many people have cut out milk and cheese—major sources of calcium. That doesn't mean you are doomed whichever way you turn. Yogurt is a good, low-fat source of calcium. So is skim milk. And if it's fat you want to cut out, eliminate meat and butter before you drop the cheese.

III. Smoking

Smoking can only lead to heartache. Inhaled smoke increases blood pressure, frees up fatty acids to form clots, damages the linings of blood vessels. Middle-aged men who smoke face ten times the risk of a heart attack as the general population. Women who smoke face about the same risk as the average male.

The components of smoke also act synergistically with other substances like alcohol and the birth control pill—which means that when it combines with another element, it doesn't just double your risk, it multiplies it many times. Smokers on the pill have six times as great a chance of dying at any moment as nonsmokers.

However, even the heaviest smoker can reverse the ill effects in almost no time. The day after you quit, your body, luxuriating in the absence of smoke, can devote more energy to repairing damaged blood vessels. Without the carbon dioxide in smoke stealing much of the available oxygen supplies, the heart doesn't have to work as hard to deliver oxygen to all the cells.

Ten to fifteen years after quitting, your health risks are barely higher than those of someone who never smoked. We carry around inside us a body-repair shop that would be the envy of the world's finest automakers—if we'd only give it a breathing spell.

Don't fool yourself by switching brands. Unfiltered cigarettes do not pose a higher risk of coronary disease than filtered; and the new low-tar, low-nicotine versions don't seem to provide any protection either, according to studies at the Boston University School of Medicine and the University of California at San Francisco. Smokeless tobacco isn't safe either. Habitual users of snuff and chewing tobacco develop the same blood levels of nicotine and cotinine (a breakdown product of nicotine) as smokers.

IV. Exercise

Regular exercise can lower blood pressure and cholesterol, increase lung capacity—one of the most important indicators of long life—minimize Type A impulses, help you lose weight. In short, it can reduce heart attacks.

One of the first studies in this area was done in England. It showed that bus conductors, who run up and down London's double-decker buses collecting fares, had less coronary heart disease than the bus drivers. Similar studies have shown that mailmen—who deliver in rain, sleet, or hail—have less heart disease than postal clerks.

A Seattle study found that men who jogged, chopped wood, or played singles tennis had lower risk for sudden heart attack than those who preferred just sitting and watching their neighbors work out.

Men active on the job, burning 600 to 1000 calories a day as farmworkers or railroad men once did, were found in past studies to postpone heart disease by ten to fifteen years longer than inactive men.

Even burning 300 calories a day by taking a brisk, hour-long walk has been shown to lower heart attack risks markedly.

Few of us can change jobs just to gain more activity. And it wouldn't do much good anyway. Today most jobs are so automated that little more than our fingers get to do any walking.

Fortunately, we don't need to get exercise through work—as long as we play. Exercise in leisure time offers even more protection than exercise on the job—three times as much, according to a New York study.

Even modest activities—walks around the neighborhood, gardening in the backyard, cleaning house enthusiastically—if done regularly, can add ten healthy years to your life. A British study found that weekend exercise alone could also ward off heart attacks.

Moderate exercise can raise the blood levels of HDL, the "good" cholesterol, and lower the "bad," LDL. (See chapter 11 on exercise for more specific details.) It can actually widen coronary arteries and lower blood pressure more effectively for some hypertensives than medication.

And those who exercise and do still have heart attacks tend to suffer milder attacks than their sedentary counterparts.

V. Diabetes

Those with diabetes are at greater risk for heart disease. But as you will see in chapter 8 on diabetes, for the vast majority who develop diabetes late in life (not in childhood), there is a great deal you can do by yourself—without drugs or insulin—to improve or eliminate this disease. The first step is to lose weight and begin exercising. These two steps alone can make your cells more receptive to insulin and eliminate the need for any external supply.

VI. The Pill

The contraceptive pill has ridden waves of good, then bad, then good reports. While excellent at preventing pregnancy, and even protective against certain types of cancer, the pill doesn't do so well for your heart.

It can drive blood pressure up in certain women. It may take six months before pressure climbs, so if you're on the pill and concerned, check your blood pressure regularly. Women on the pill also have 6 times the normal risk of stroke; 2.8 times greater chance of heart attack if you're between 30 and 40; 4.7 times greater if you're over 40.

And if you smoke at the same time, your risk rockets to 20 times greater for stroke, 10 times greater for heart attack.

VII. Meditation or Relaxation Therapy

The calming relaxation techniques that the religious and secular alike have been using for millennia can lower blood pressure. Meditators have been shown to lower their blood pressure from an average of 146/92 to 135/87 in twenty weeks. Relaxation exercises also reduce heart rate and breathing while not altering the oxygen supplies in the bloodstream. In short, relaxation techniques can reverse many of the bodily changes that stress brings about.

VIII. The Good, the Bad, and the Doubtful

ASPIRIN

An aspirin a day may be better than an apple—for men with heart problems. Then again, it may not.

Four studies have indicated that for men regular doses of aspirin reduced heart attacks by 25 to 65 percent. However, a fifth study—the largest one of all—did not find any confirmation of this link.

Aspirin's virtue (aside from its painkilling powers) is that it has anticlotting properties that may reduce the atherosclerosis and blood clotting that lead to heart attacks. While cardiologists admit that they don't know if taking two or three aspirins a day will help, many confide that they take them anyway, if they are more at risk for heart disease than ulcers.

As for women, the benefits seem remote. A 1982 Boston study found that aspirin did not protect women under fifty against a first heart attack. So for now, at least, women should save aspirin for a headache.

SZECHUAN FOOD

The Chinese black tree fungus (mu-er), a mushroom used in southern Chinese cooking, inhibits platelet function and thus might ultimately inhibit heart disease, according to research at the University of Minnesota's School of Medicine. Platelets are small cells in the blood that aside from serving us well by stopping bleeding and causing clotting also serve us ill when they add to the hardening of the arteries that leads to heart disease. Use of this mushroom may help explain why the Chinese—and especially the southern Chinese—have a very low incidence of heart disease despite high sodium intakes and high hypertension levels. Onion and garlic, heavily present in this diet, may also have a similar antiplatelet effect. (Aspirin, too, seems to denature platelets.)

The evidence so far is not conclusive. But a Szechuan meal now and again can't hurt.

BREAKFAST

Not eating breakfast has even been fingered as a hypertension culprit. In a study of 1500 children, aged nine to thirteen, a food science professor at Clemson University found that those who regularly eat breakfast are less likely to have high blood pressure than those who rush off on an empty stomach. Whether the issue is really that breakfast foods provide some chemical protection or that people who eat breakfast routinely are more likely to come from stable homes where nutrition is regarded as important (and for that reason are less prone to hypertension) remains a subject for further study. In the meantime, sit down and eat your yogurt.

SELENIUM

This mineral, receiving even more attention as a cancer deterrent, seems to be linked to warding off heart disease as well. In places where the mineral is found in high concentrations in the soil and thus in the water supply and the foods grown, such as Colorado Springs, the death rate from heart disease is 67 percent lower than the national average. In a city such as Washington, D.C. (densely populated areas seem to be low in selenium), for example, the heart disease death rate is 22 percent above the national average. (For a list of foods high in this mineral, turn to chapter 7, "Cancer.")

Taking much higher doses of selenium than the federal government's RDA (recommended daily allowance) may be riskier than having low levels of selenium. However, ensuring that you get an adequate supply would also be prudent.

SOFT WATER, SOFT DATA

People in areas with soft water have higher heart attack rates, according to a study of 575 communities in Canada. The explanation may be that soft water lacks magnesium; animals with a magnesium deficiency tend to develop irregular heartbeats. So far, in people, this is not considered a serious risk factor.

IX. A Word on Drugs

Drug therapy is often prescribed for hypertension and can work. If a doctor prescribes medication, and you have carefully discussed the pros and cons with him or her and no other changes in weight, diet, or relaxation seem to help, then you should follow the prescribed regimen.

Many people, however, do not. Among those advised to take drugs, one study found only 50 to 60 percent took their pills. Doctors should note that patients asked to take an active role in their own therapy—taking their own blood pressure and charting their progress—not only complied more with the doctor's prescription but lowered their blood pressure.

The drugs commonly used do not unclog arteries, but they have been shown to reduce deaths from heart attacks and strokes substantially (in one study by nearly one-half)—and improve the conditions of those with only mild hypertension as well. It also must be added that most drugs used are relatively new—introduced well after 1950, so all the long-term side effects are not fully known.

Beta blockers are the leaders among these "new" drugs that look especially promising for preventing subsequent heart attacks in those who have already suffered one. Within six months of having a heart attack, your chances for a second are four to eight times as great as the average person. A controlled, double-blind study (the Rolls-Royce of scientific methods—reliable, respected, and expensive) of 3937 people who had survived a heart attack, half of whom were given the beta blocker Inderal, found that those taking the drug had 26 percent fewer deaths.

The efficacy of the beta blocker was so unquestionable, according to the researchers, that they stopped the experiment nine months earlier than scheduled. They didn't think it was fair to keep the control group from sharing in the benefits, too.

While beta blockers are not yet being prescribed for prevention of a first heart attack, many are exploring whether that might be advisable. Work is also being done to see if they may be useful in modifying Type A behavior because they block production of norepinephrine. Currently the only people with no specific disease history using the drug are performers—actors and musicians—who are using beta blockers to reduce the anxiety of stage fright.

But for now, the only sure methods for preventing heart attacks and strokes lie in our behavior, not in drugs. And this is behavior we can control.

SUMMARY: HOW TO PREVENT HEART DISEASE

Know your risks—and reduce the ones you can.

Each small change you can make lowers your risk.

But it also works the other way around—in spades. Each additional risk factor more than adds to, it *multiplies* your heart trouble. For example, if you smoke a pack a day and also have slightly high cholesterol levels (10 to 15 percent above normal), then you have three times the average risk of suffering a heart attack or stroke. Someone who adds high blood pressure to the smoking and cholesterol record faces five times the chances of a heart attack and more than ten times the risk of a stroke.

It's never too late—or too early—to begin making changes.

Risk Factors Summarized

1. Age—Risk rises with age.
2. Sex—Men have higher risks.
3. Race—Blacks have higher risks.
4. Family history—Blood relatives of those who have died early of heart disease are considered to be at higher risk.
5. Blood pressure—The lower the better.
6. Cholesterol levels—The lower the better.
7. Blood sugar—High levels, indicating diabetes, increase the risk.
8. Smoking—The more cigarettes, the higher the risk.
9. Type A behavior—These learned reactions to stress pose as serious a risk as smoking or having high cholesterol.
10. Overweight—Too much food, usually of the wrong kind, raises risks.

Ways to Reduce the Risks Summarized

1. Modify your time-pressured, angry Type A behavior. You weren't born a Type A and you don't have to stay that way.
2. Take your diet seriously, or it will take you seriously by surprise.

• Cut down on fats, especially saturated fats, by eating less red meat and more fish, chicken, and low-fat dairy products. This will help not simply to lower total cholesterol levels in the blood but also, more important, to raise the ratio of HDL to LDL.

• Eat more fruits and vegetables, especially those rich in B-6, which may further lower blood cholesterol levels.

• Step up calcium consumption, to lower blood pressure, by eating more yogurt, skim milk, and low-fat cheeses.

• Stop shaking the salt—most of us eat ten times the amount we need every day. And high salt intake raises blood pressure.

• Lose weight if you're more than 20 percent over your "ideal" weight. For every pound of fat, the body needs about three-quarters of a mile of blood vessels to feed and keep it going. So, if you are 20 pounds overweight, your heart has to work overtime pushing blood through 15 extra miles of pipes—and as the blood makes a complete circulation every 13 seconds, that means over 4000 extra miles every hour, 24 hours a day, 365 days a year. Not surprising, then, that extra weight raises blood pressure and adds to the strain on your heart.

3. Go easy on the alcohol. A drink or two is probably not a hazard to your heart, but it can put you at risk in other ways (car accidents, cancer vulnerability) that could strain your heart and the rest of you as well.

4. Cutting back on caffeine may not only lower blood pressure but cholesterol as well.

5. Exercise—get out there and get the old bones moving—three times a week. Jogging is not required; in fact it's not even the best exercise for most of us. Just start small and eventually work up a sweat. It may raise your cleaning bills but it will lower your risks for heart attack and strokes.

6. Smoking—don't bother fighting or switching. No new brand, no filter, no vitamin or wonder drug can erase the damage smoking does to your heart and blood vessels. You want to come a long way, baby? Quit.

7. Learn how to cope with stress and use it to your advantage.

For the step-by-step specifics on how to go about incorporating all of these changes into your daily life to prevent heart troubles, turn to chapters 10 through 17.

But for safety, just in case you may have already pushed too hard, too long, it is important to acquaint yourself with the early-warning signs of heart trouble and the procedure to follow in an emergency.

Stroke Symptoms

These symptoms of a "temporary stroke" or TIA (transient ischemic attack) are similar to a full-fledged stroke—but they last only minutes or hours—not a lifetime. Recognizing them is your chance to save yourself before suffering the devastating effects of a genuine stroke.

1. Numbness or tingling in one side of the face or body.
2. Weakness or paralysis (you may act clumsy) in limbs on one side.
3. Blurriness of vision, confusion, dizziness.
4. Difficulty speaking or swallowing.
5. Sudden headache or seizures when there is no history of them.

What to Do

You can wait for a few hours or days, but as soon as possible report your symptoms to a doctor who will determine if anticoagulants or other treatment is called for.

Angina Symptoms

Angina pectoris, which means "strangulation of the breastbone," refers to a pain that occurs when the heart is not getting quite enough oxygen and blood—a condition more common in women than men.

1. The chest pain is characterized by heavy pressure or a squeezing sensation directly under the breastbone. The pain of angina pectoris is brief—usually no more than 10 minutes.
2. The pain can occur as a result of emotional or physical exertion.
3. If the pain does not stop upon resting or goes on longer than 10 minutes, the problem may not be angina but a heart attack.

What to Do

See a doctor as soon as possible. Nitroglycerin, often prescribed, can increase the blood flow to the heart temporarily and relieve angina within 5 minutes. If nitroglycerin does not work during an angina attack, you may be having a heart attack and should get to a hospital immediately.

Heart Attack Symptoms

1. An uncomfortable pressure or squeezing sensation in the center of the chest that may extend up into the neck and jaw, often radiating into the left arm (though the right or both may be involved).
2. The pain is rarely a sharp, stabbing pain and is rarely below the nipple or to the left of the heart.
3. The pain usually lasts at least 5 or 10 minutes, though in rare cases it may come and go, and is no better when you lie down.
4. Dizziness, sweating, nausea, or shortness of breath may accompany the pain.
5. Not all of these symptoms need occur together.

What to Do

Get to a hospital quickly, even if the pain doesn't seem crippling. Most heart attack victims die in the first two hours after an attack. Calling a friend to drive you is usually faster than waiting for an ambulance. If your community has a mobile coronary care unit, call that first.

If you know you are at risk, make sure someone else in the house learns how to administer CPR (cardiopulmonary resuscitation). If you have a sudden heart attack and are not breathing or displaying a pulse, someone else must perform cardiovascular pulmonary resuscitation (CPR) on the way to the hospital. (See chapter 17 for instruction on the technique.)

7
Cancer

EVEN THE SANEST and calmest among us seem to lose composure when the subject turns to cancer. The fear is deep but unspoken: if my number's up, my number's up, and there's nothing I can do.

At first glance, the statistics seem to support such an attitude. Sooner or later, at the current rates of incidence, nearly one in three of us will develop cancer in our lifetime. Over 5 million Americans alive today have been diagnosed as having cancer—over 850,000 people will be diagnosed this year with the disease. Close to 500,000 will die this year from the disease that Americans fear more than any other.

But this need not be the case.

We could prevent anywhere from 35 to 80 percent of all cancers right now, this very minute, without scientists' going one step further to pierce the mysteries of this complex disease. That means that anywhere from 165,000 to 400,000 lives might be saved a year, simply by changing smoking, drinking, eating, and exercising habits.

Unfortunately, too many of us allow our action and inaction to be guided by the myths that invariably sprout up around fearful subjects. We are not drowning in a sea of carcinogens, and everything will not cause cancer if taken in large enough doses—two notions that have taken root in the public imagination. Very few substances actually cause cancer. The major cancer threats today stem from things that we can still control.

Causes and Cures

Cancer does not usually pounce upon us suddenly. Most often it comes after decades of subtle bodily abuse and exposure to risks. The direct cause may be certain chemicals, viruses, even a gene within us all from birth, dubbed an "oncogene," that somehow gets turned on by mistake and causes cancer. But the most common factor is that our immune system has weakened—from not taking care of ourselves, our diet, from age, stress, cigarettes, and the like—and it can no longer prevent the cancer cells from growing out of control.

There are always a few cells among the body's trillions going out of control. Our immune system, working like a bouncer at a nightclub, silently ejects these troublemakers before they can clump together into an obstreperous tumor. But when the immune system begins to falter—a process that occurs with age but can be speeded up or slowed down by how we behave—then the intruders run free, and we are more likely to become cancer patients.

Because cancer is not one disease but hundreds, and because even the same type of cancer will behave very differently in different people, we cannot expect that there will ever be one drug or one vaccine to wipe it out. The overall death rate for cancer has not changed significantly in the last fifty years. Advances in treatments are coming slowly, and even "cures" that prolong life for five or ten more years do so only with a great deal of pain and suffering.

Few of us appreciate the extent to which the current "cures"—the radiation, the chemotherapy—while getting all the credit, are merely sidekicks to our immune system. They cannot get rid of all the cancer cells, though they destroy a good number. What the drugs are really doing is giving the immune system a boost. Actually it is we, in the end—through our killer T-lymphocytes—who must search out and destroy every last one of those cancer cells if we are to survive. And thus, real cure depends not so much on those aids—though they are not to be taken for granted—but upon the health of our own systems. The best chemicals can do nothing, not one thing, if our immune systems do not take up the major cancer-controlling role.

For those of us alive now, the one in three who could be headed for trouble, our best hope for staying alive is prevention of cancer, not cure. And it is through achieving optimum health that we keep our immune system—our selves—in prime condition.

How Much Is Preventable?

Cancer epidemiologists, who track the causes of diseases, have made the following estimates on which factors play the critical preventive roles.

- Diet changes might reduce cancers by 35 percent.
- Stopping smoking could save perhaps 75 to 90 percent of those who die of lung cancer and reduce cancer overall by 30 percent. (Lung cancer rates for women have tripled since 1964.)
- Alcohol may contribute to 3 percent of cancers.
- Air pollution may account for 1 to 2 percent.
- Industrial chemicals leading to occupational hazards are thought to cause less than 1 percent.
- Staying out of the sun might save as many as 5000 lives, or 1 percent of cancer deaths.
- Medicines and procedures, including X rays, may cause 1 percent.
- Early detection of breast cancer, which could be possible with more frequent self-examinations and professional examinations, could save up to 25 percent of the over 30,000 women who die of this disease every year.

This does not mean that a cancer patient is to blame for his or her disease. There are factors beyond our control. Aside from the elusive contributions of heredity and chance, there is no denying that dangerous pollutants in the air, water, and at the workplace can put some in jeopardy.

Those who work in the rubber industry have a high incidence of bladder cancer; uranium and other miners bear high lung cancer risks along with those in the steel industry exposed to the coke ovens. Some diseases (asbestosis, pleural and peritoneal mesothelioma) never occur except in those exposed to asbestos.

But we must also face the fact that our actions—or inactions—can make our chances for health better or worse. Asbestos alone has rarely led to lung cancer, but for asbestos workers who also smoke heavily, the risk for lung cancer jumps to over ninety times as high as for those who neither smoke nor handle asbestos.

Our diet, daily habits, the drugs we use—and even our personalities—all play a part in our vulnerability to a disease whose very name scares the wits out of most of us—but which can be outwitted by those who know what to do and what not to do as well.

Trends in Cancer Incidence

Fifty years ago stomach cancer was the leading cancer; lung cancer is now. Most likely there is less stomach cancer because we're consuming more foods rich in vitamin C, which seems to counteract certain cancer-causing chemicals in foods, particularly nitrates and nitrites. In Japan, stomach cancer is still the leading cancer—eight times as common as in the United States. And scientists point the accusatory finger at the Japanese diet, which tends to be low in fresh fruits and vegetables (and thus low in vitamin C) and heavily weighted in pickled and smoked fish and similarly treated vegetables (high in nitrates and nitrites which the body converts to the carcinogens nitrosamines and nitrosamides).

There is more lung cancer now—accounting for one-fourth of all cancers—for a very simple reason: we continue to smoke. Women are smoking more than ever, and lung cancer in females is up fourfold since 1964.

CANCER TREND SUMMARY
OVER THE LAST TWO DECADES

Leading cancers in men	Lung, prostate, colon, bladder, rectum, stomach, and pancreas
Leading cancers in women	Breast, colon, uterus, lung, ovary, rectum, and cervix
Going down	Stomach, liver For women, cancers of the uterus, bladder, colon, and rectum down slightly
Going up	Lung and pancreas For women, breast and ovary For men, esophagus, kidney, prostate, leukemia

CANCER DEATH RATES BY SITE—UNITED STATES, 1930–1978*

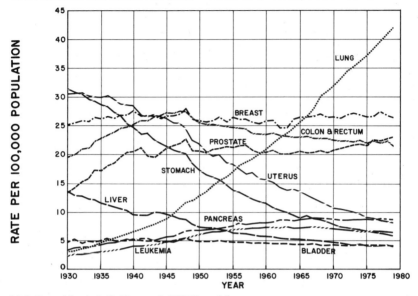

Rate for the population standardized for age on the 1970 U.S. population
Sources of Data: National Center for Health Statistics and Bureau of the Census, United States.

Note: Rates are for both sexes combined except breast and uterus female population only
and prostate male population only.

*Reprinted with permission from the American Cancer Society.

Smoking

Everyone likes to hear tales of some wizened old lady who at age ninety-three still belts down a pint of moonshine and walks three miles into town every day for her pack of cigarettes. We love it because she flies in the face of all the odds, she rises above the risks—a rare survivor.

The only trouble is for every one such cigarette-puffing miracle, there are hundreds of thousands of mere mortals—325,000 a year to be precise—who smoke and who die.

There is no question that dozens of the 2500 compounds that make up smoke irritate tissue cells and cause them to divide abnormally as cancerous cells. Smoking is linked not only to lung cancer but to cancers of the mouth, lip, esophagus, larynx, pharynx, pancreas, bladder, in addition to heart disease, chronic bronchitis, emphysema, flu, and stomach ulcers.

If smoking were eliminated, so would 85 to 95 percent of all respiratory cancers, and other cancers, too—perhaps 150,000 lives a year could be saved. And once you get lung cancer, the prognosis is not a cheery one. After a conclusive diagnosis, 70 percent die within a year; only 9 percent live for five years after the diagnosis.

If you're ready to pack up your cigarette packs, turn to chapter 16 for a rundown on the best techniques for quitting.

What to Do If You Can't Quit Yet

If you're not quite ready yet, here are some things you should know to reduce your risk in the meantime.

Smoking is not an all-or-nothing proposition—you are not simply a smoker or a nonsmoker. Your risk rises—and lowers—in proportion to the number of cigarettes smoked and how deeply you inhale.

Just hanging around smokers can increase your risks. Nonsmokers whose spouses smoke more than a pack a day have double the risk of dying of lung cancer as people whose spouses do not smoke. And if you work in the same room with smokers, you'll end up after twenty years with as much respiratory damage as if you were smoking a little more than half a pack a day—even if a cigarette never directly touched your lips. Naturally, the risk goes way up for smokers sitting in smoke-filled rooms, too. Sidestream or secondhand smoke contains many of the same pollutants as directly inhaled smoke—some (including nicotine, tar, aniline, nitrosamine) in even more dangerous concentrations.

So if you must smoke, do it only in a ventilated place—never in an enclosed compartment like an elevator, or a car or train with the windows closed. In the house, get one of those ashtrays that filters the smoke immediately.

Low-tar and nicotine cigarettes are not likely to be any safer than any other cigarettes. People tend to smoke more of and inhale more deeply on the "low-tars" until they often wind up doing as much damage as those smoking even nonfiltered brands.

And switching to little cigars instead of cigarettes may be even worse. They have more tar and nicotine than cigarettes, four to eight times the nitrogen compounds which play a role in carcinogenesis, and two to three times the carbon monoxide levels.

Eating carefully is especially critical for smokers. Smoke destroys vitamin C in the body. So not only do you lose a critical vitamin, but you lose its additional cancer-protection powers. If you must puff, keep a fruit bowl next to your cigarette pack.

Don't smoke in front of your children. As a short-term danger, children are more vulnerable to air pollutants like smoke because they have greater breathing capacity for their body weight than adults and will take in a disproportionate share of the noxious fumes. In the long run, there is an even greater risk—that the child will follow your example. If children do not see their parents smoke, and few of their friends smoke, the vast majority will not smoke. Unfortunately, the reverse holds true, too; if they see you smoke, they will copy. And the earlier they start, the more likely they are to be hooked for life.

Diet and Cancer

Diet may be responsible for 40 percent of cancers in men and 60 percent of cancers in women.

Individual foods do not usually act suddenly to trigger cancer so much as they either promote or inhibit the growth of tumors. It is a process that takes place over a period of years—from a stage when cancerous cells are few and easily handled to the point at which they grow into trouble.

Total Calories—"Enough" Is Too Much

The major problem with most of our diets is that we eat too much. Animals fed on restricted diets—for example, rats fed healthy diets one day and made to fast each alternate day—live longer and have lower incidence of tumors.

Will it work for humans? It's hard to say. We do know that being overweight seems to have the opposite effect—shorter life and higher risk that tumors will develop. Though the researchers who did these rodent studies are not yet willing to make recommendations for humans, several admit privately that they think the implications look promising enough to cut back on their food intake and even try fasting one day a week.

And it's never too late to start. Even rats put on this restricted diet in what would be the equivalent of middle age live longer than average.

Fats

Fats spell trouble. Consuming as much fat as Americans typically do has been linked to the high incidence of breast, prostate, and colon cancer. Japanese women, who have a much lower-fat diet and less incidence of breast cancer, become more susceptible to breast cancer when they move to America and adopt the diet here. Their daughters have just about as high a risk as their American peers. For Japanese men who come to America, it doesn't even take a generation for them to lose their protection against colon cancer; as soon as they adopt the Western diet their risk shoots up nearly as high as that of American men.

And the culprit seems to be all fat—not just saturated (animal) fats which pose dangers for heart disease, but polyunsaturated (vegetable) fats as well. Colon cancer rates have remained constant despite the rise in the proportion of polyunsaturated fats in Americans' diets over the last twenty years.

No one is entirely certain how fats work against us. But one hypothesis is that fats and cholesterol, in addition to clogging up the arterial works and posing a threat of heart disease, lead to a kind of clogging in the digestive system as well. Fatty foods take longer to digest than carbohydrates and stay longer in the colon as waste, too. The bacteria that live in the colon break down these wastes into substances that may be carcinogenic—and the longer the waste stays there, the longer the colon is exposed to these noxious chemicals.

Another hypothesis is that intestinal bacteria, working on cholesterol, can also produce a substance very similar to the female sex hormone, estrogen, which may trigger the growth of cancers in the breast and uterus. Researchers at Tufts University of Medicine have found that vegetarian women (whose diets are low in fats and high in fiber) produce less estrogen than nonvegetarian and obese women and excrete more of it—they also have a lower than average incidence of breast cancer.

Proteins

High intake of proteins, too, seems to promote tumors, but the research in this area is not yet as extensive as that for fats. It also may be that those populations studied which eat too much protein get much of that protein from meat or other fatty sources, thereby confusing the issue. So far the research waters here are about as clear as unstrained chicken soup.

Fruits and Vegetables—Fiber, Folic Acid and Vitamins A, C, and E

Fruits and vegetables seem to inhibit cancers of the breast, colon, and prostate. The virtues of these humble foods seem to lie in their high fiber content and their vitamins.

Fiber-rich foods provide the bulk that speeds food through the system, thus flushing the digestive passageways and making sure the bacteria get the shortest time to do their cancer-conversion work.

Folic acid, one of the B-complex vitamins, seems to be showing promising signs in preventing cervical cancer. Foods rich in folic acid include kidney, liver, yeast, and green leafy vegetables.

But even more important, according to a report by the National Academy of Science's National Research Council, seem to be vitamins A and C (perhaps E, too) as well as the mineral selenium.

Vitamin A. Vitamin A has been shown to inhibit cancers of the breast, urinary bladder, skin, and lung in animals. Vitamin A is critical for the normal growth of cells on the skin and lining of most of our internal organs.

For those who smoke, vitamin A may be even more critical. Smokers who eat large amounts of carrots, spinach, and other vegetables high in vitamin A, have less risk of lung cancer than typical smokers, according to a Chicago study of nearly 2000 men.

For those who already have cancer, this vitamin also may make chemotherapy and radiation treatment more effective and prolong the life-span. It may also prevent recurrences of the disease after surgery, as high doses of synthetic A did with skin cancer in a study at the University of Arizona Cancer Center in Tucson.

However, this does not mean we should all go and load up on vitamin supplements. Vitamin A in large doses (from vitamin pills) can have dangerous side effects. The only safe path is eating foods high in vitamin A and beta-carotene (a protovitamin from plants that the body converts to vitamin A.)

Foods rich in vitamin A include deep yellow fruits and vegetables and dark green vegetables—particularly broccoli, brussels sprouts, cabbage, carrots, cauliflower, collards, kale, mustard greens, pumpkins, spinach, sweet potatoes, turnip greens, and winter squash—as well as chick-peas, cereal grains, dried beans, soybeans, liver, eggs, milk, butter, and fish-liver oils.

Fish-liver oils? Yes. Remember not so long ago when mothers used to give their children a daily swallow of cod-liver oil? They knew, as "old wives" often do, that this foul-smelling potion had to be good for you. It is a rich and especially safe source of vitamin A for children, as the chances of their overdoing are slim. Other fish oils, especially halibut and shark, contain good supplies of vitamin A and are available in pill form. Though high-potency pills are sold, anyone considering any higher doses than 10,000 units should consult a doctor. The recommended daily allowance for men is 5000 IUs (international units) and for women 4000 IUs.

Cabbage, broccoli, cauliflower, and brussels sprouts, in addition to their vitamin A, also contain something called "indoles," which have been shown to inhibit tumor growth in mice and rats. Patients with colon and rectal cancer have been found to have diets very low in these vegetables.

Vitamin C. Vitamin C inhibits the formation of cancerous compounds—nitrosamines or nitrosamides—in our digestive systems. These dangerous compounds can arise as we digest foods with nitrates and nitrites, substances which exist naturally in many foods and are also added as a preservative to cured meats, including hot dogs, bacon, bologna, salami, and other luncheon meats. However, if vitamin C is present, it competes with the "amine" or "amide" to latch up with the nitrosating agent. If the vitamin wins, so do we, for no nitrosamine or nitrosamide is formed.

Consuming at least 90 milligrams a day of vitamin C may help prevent cervical cancer, according to research conducted at the Albert Einstein College of Medicine, in New York. It may also protect against cancers of the lung, skin, colon, and stomach. And a study at Memorial Sloan-Kettering Cancer Center, in New York, suggests it may also prevent the development of polyps that are linked to rectal or colon cancer.

Vitamin C is an antioxidant, which means, according to the "free radical" theory of cancer causation, that it can prevent the conversion of many other chemicals into active carcinogens after they've been eaten or inhaled. (For those interested in a brief outline, free radicals are cells that are missing an electron—these result when oxygen combines with an atom and knocks off an electron—a normal process of living, breathing, and aging. Free radicals are thought to seek out their missing electrons and thereby set off a chain reaction creating more cells deficient in an electron that can lead to cell damage typical of aging.)

If you want to help lower your chances for cancer of the stomach and esophagus especially, either steer clear of smoke-cured meats and pickled foods, or at least make sure to have a glass of fruit juice before the meal, or a vegetable or fruit salad and a potato on the side.

Foods high in vitamin C include citrus fruits, strawberries, cantaloupe, tomatoes, potatoes, cabbage, broccoli, kale, green peppers.

Vitamin E. Vitamin E, also an antioxidant, does much the same thing as vitamin C, in test tube studies. However, the research on this vitamin is not as far along as for vitamin C.

Foods rich in vitamin E are green vegetables, eggs, wheat germ oil, vegetable oils (especially soybean, corn and cottonseed), nuts, legumes, oatmeal, and organ meats such as liver and kidneys.

Minerals

Selenium. This mineral has been touted as a cancer wonder drug by many overly enthusiastic health-food aficionados. The evidence so far can support only considerably more reserved acclaim. Epidemiologists have found that people living in areas where (because of the soil content) the per capita consumption of selenium is high have a lower incidence of colon, rectal and breast cancer (and heart disease, too). In one study, 80 percent of laboratory mice who were exposed to cancer-causing viruses and chemicals and who were also given selenium in their drinking water did not get cancer.

Soil and water supplies in the densely populated areas of the Northeast and North Central United States, in particular Massachusetts and New York, are generally lowest in selenium. The wide-open spaces of North Dakota and Colorado, however, have quite high levels.

But again, taking supplements in pill form is risky. High dosages can be dangerous. And, according to the National Academy of Sciences, there is no proof that swallowing supplements beyond the 200 micrograms that most of us should get in a balanced daily diet will do any good.

The best food sources for selenium are fish (especially tuna and herring), seaweed, organ meats such as liver and kidneys, brewer's yeast, bran, broccoli, wheat germ, whole grains, poultry and a number of other fruits and vegetables.

Iron. Deficiencies of iron can increase the risk of Plummer-Vinson syndrome, which is linked to cancer of the upper alimentary tract. This deficiency may also be related to gastric cancer. For many Americans, especially women, who do not get enough iron in their diets, multivitamins with added iron cannot hurt. Foods rich in iron are eggs, fish, poultry, meats (especially organ meats), green leafy vegetables, and dried fruits.

Copper, zinc, molybdenum, and iodine. All of these may inhibit tumor growth; however, test results are inconclusive so far. Studies abroad have shown that while molybdenum may inhibit tumors in the esophagus and stomach, both too little and too much iodine have been linked to thyroid cancer.

Arsenic, cadmium, and lead. Dangerous minerals. Too much can encourage tumor growth. However, the normal range of the American diet rarely contains dangerous levels.

Alcohol

Heavy drinking may increase the chances of getting mouth and throat cancer anywhere from two to six times above average. It also heightens the risk of cancers of the esophagus, larynx, and liver. Heavy beer drinking has been linked to cancers of the colon and rectum.

Liquor also acts synergistically with cigarette smoke—that means that the combination multiplies the risk many times higher than if the two risk levels were simply added together. Drinking and smoking considerably raise one's chances for cancers of the mouth, larynx, esophagus, and respiratory tract.

Caffeine

Caffeine has brought mixed reports. Though at least one study links coffee and tea drinking to pancreatic cancer, others find no ties. When people put milk in their tea, as the English routinely do, the cancer dangers seem even more remote as the milk seems to bind up the tannins and prevent their ill effects.

Many people find that consuming caffeine increases their desire for alcohol and sometimes cigarettes. Whether the desire stems from trying to soothe caffeine jitters or something chemically subtler, the dangers of alcohol and cigarettes are well documented.

Food Additives

Additives have become a dirty word. We think of all sorts of nasty chemicals that must be doing us in. And indeed cyclamates, red dye No. 2, diethylstilbestrol (DES), formerly used in the feed of chicken and cattle, have been banned.

But a few additives may even prove helpful in the fight against cancer. BHA (butylated hydroxyanisol), an antioxidant added to cooking oils, bakery products, even to drugs to keep them fresh, behaves much as the other antioxidants, vitamins E and C, do, in inhibiting cancer growth. (The subject is under investigation at Johns Hopkins University.)

However, that doesn't mean one should become blasé about devouring processed foods laden with additives. There are also 12,000 other chemicals indirectly added to foods—many used in food packaging that seeps into the foods, such as vinyl chloride and acrylonitrile—that have not been tested and proved safe.

Saccharin

The 1977 battle to ban this synthetic white powder five hundred times sweeter than sugar was lost, but the battle cries of the warriors still echo. The National Academy of Sciences warns that however "weak" a carcinogen, it still has the potential to increase your cancer risk. The American Cancer Society argues that there was "no evidence that it is carcinogenic in humans. And it is of great value in dietetic food used to control diabetes and obesity."

However, saccharin did cause cancer in lab rats. True, the rats were given higher doses than the thirstiest diet-soda drinker would likely consume. But even though many innocuous substances when given in unusually high doses can suddenly become lethal (examples of salt and arsenic, found naturally in certain vegetables, come to mind), only very few substances—no matter what the dosage—will become carcinogenic.

The question remains: if saccharin causes cancer in high doses, what will it do in smaller doses? For now, this substance remains not only in diet drinks but in toothpastes, mouthwashes, and some six hundred medicines from antacids to chewable vitamins. You must weigh its potential cancer risks against the obesity risks, such as they are, in consuming the seventeen calories in a teaspoon of sugar.

Cook and Handle It Right

Not only what you eat but also the way you cook it can affect cancer risks. Frying meats at a high heat, over 300 degrees, produces mutagens. Broiling does the same, and charcoal broiling, sad to say, is the worst in terms of increasing the formation of cancer-causing elements.

It's better to cook those burgers slowly, or sear both sides at a high heat briefly and then continue the cooking process at a lower heat. Eating meat rare can reduce your risk by 90 percent.

If you can't resist the charcoal grill occasionally, at least make sure to eat a big fresh salad of lettuce (romaine has twice the vitamin C of iceberg lettuce and four times the vitamin A) and tomatoes along with it. And to play it really safe, have fruit salad for dessert—also rich in protective vitamin C.

Don't cut up fruits and vegetables and leave them exposed to the light and air long before eating—they lose vitamin C. A sliced cucumber loses one-third of its vitamin C in an hour, half in four hours.

Even uncut fruits and vegetables need to be refrigerated. While it may look pretty to keep them in a bowl on the table as a centerpiece, they lose 25 percent of their vitamin C in 72 hours at room temperature while losing only 10 percent in 96 hours in the fridge.

As for juices, it is best to buy them in opaque containers. Those in glass containers that sit on the grocer's shelves exposed to fluorescent lights may have lost some of their nutritional value. Keep juice covered tightly and make it in quantities that will be consumed in a couple of days.

Don't soak vegetables in liquid either before or during cooking as it will leach the water-soluble B-complex and C vitamins right out. If you use all the liquid ultimately to make a soup or a sauce, this cooking method is acceptable. Otherwise, you'd be better off steaming or stir-frying vegetables.

Summary: General Cancer-Prevention Diet

What's a hungry person to do? What's safe and what isn't?

Here's a general rundown to keep in mind when looking over your diet. (For tips on satisfying substitutes for your present habits, turn to chapter 15 on diet.) You can't avoid everything or include everything—but the more you do the better off you'll be.

Eat

- More fish and chicken instead of red meat—fish is not only low in fat but high in selenium.

- Skim versions of dairy products—they usually have all the nutritional advantages of their whole-milk counterparts—just less fat. Skim milk, cheese made from skim milk, and yogurt are all good sources of vitamin A.
- Citrus fruits—they're especially high in vitamin C.
- Dark green vegetables—especially broccoli, spinach, kale, along with mustard, turnip, and collard greens—are high in vitamin A.
- Deep yellow vegetables—carrots, sweet potatoes and squash are especially rich in vitamin A.
- Foods rich in both vitamin A and vitamin C—potatoes, tomatoes, peppers, brussels sprouts, and cauliflower (in addition to the vegetables listed above).
- Fiber-rich foods—vegetables, fruits, and whole-grain breads, and brown rice are beneficial not only for their vitamins and minerals but their fiber content, too.

Avoid

- Fatty meats.
- Both saturated and polyunsaturated fats—cut back on both butter and margarine, and on salad oils.
- Large quantities of dairy products, especially whole-milk products.
- Salt-cured, pickled, and smoked foods—including hot dogs, sausages, bologna, ham. You might have to try that bagel without any lox.
- Alcohol in large quantities—more than two or three drinks a day.
- Caffeine in large quantities—more than two or three cups of coffee, tea, or cola a day.

The Pill—Back in Good Graces?

The pill has changed since its introduction in the 1960s, and so has its reputation very recently. First embraced as the dream contraceptive, then shunned and feared as a possible cause of cancer and heart disease, it has now been largely vindicated as far as cancer is concerned. While it still may pose added risks for cardiovascular problems among some, the evidence is mounting that it can actually provide a great deal of protection against certain cancers and other conditions.

Cancer of the ovary and uterus. There is consistent evidence that pill use reduces the risk of these two cancers by about half. The Centers for Disease Control in Atlanta estimates that it may prevent four thousand cases of these two cancers yearly. Women receive this protective effect if they took the pill for at least a year, and the benefits persist for at least ten years after stopping contraceptive use.

Breast cancer. The latest data suggest the pill does not increase breast cancer risk as once feared. And a Scandinavian study found that pill users who contracted this disease had higher chances of survival than nonusers.

Pelvic inflammatory disease (PID). Pill users develop one-third to one-half the rate of this infection of the reproductive tract as nonusers. PID is not only painful, it can lead to infertility.

Toxic-shock syndrome. No one knows why, but pill users seem to have one-fourth the risk.

Rheumatoid arthritis. Pill use and pregnancy—both of which increase female hormones—protect against this type of arthritis and may explain why this disease (which affects about 2 percent of all women) has declined among women since the 1960s.

Today's pill contains a combination of estrogen and progestin. In the early days many pills were sequential, giving first one then the other. New pills also contain much lower doses of these hormones—as little as one-tenth of the older versions.

However, the pill is not advisable for women over thirty-five since it can increase cardiovascular problems (heart attacks and strokes) which women become increasingly susceptible to as they age. And it is not a good contraceptive at any age for those who smoke, as this heightens the cardiovascular risk.

Estrogen alone—prescribed for middle-aged women to alleviate unpleasant symptoms of menopause—still is considered risky. It seems to increase the chances of developing uterine cancer.

What Else Should We Avoid?

ULTRAVIOLET (UV) LIGHT—BUT NOT ALL THE TIME

Cultivating a tan may turn out to *look* healthier than it really is. Sunlight and X rays are associated with free radical reactions that can alter the cell's DNA and lead to skin cancer.

Malignant melanoma, a type of skin cancer on the rise, usually starts in a mole and then spreads to lymph nodes in the armpits, neck, and groin. If the disease is caught early, the outlook can be good. Otherwise, it spreads, resisting chemotherapy.

The ultraviolet (UV) radiation in natural sunlight may also inhibit the immune system's ability to challenge growing tumors. The best bet is to avoid the summer midday sun, when UV light is strongest, even in cloudy or rainy weather. And if you stay out, use sunscreens (containing PABA) that actually block UV light.

However, you shouldn't avoid sunlight altogether. Unless you're at particularly high risk for skin cancer, some exposure to natural sunlight is essential to good health. Our bodies need sun in order to synthesize vitamin D (that's why it's known as "the sunshine vitamin"). Staying inside with only artificial light can make us vulnerable to eye diseases, hypertension, even arthritis. Light waves absorbed through the eye may stimulate the pituitary gland which in turn stimulates the neuroendocrine system and the production of hormones. Glass and plastic—from a window or even eyeglasses and sunglasses—block UV light and that needed stimulation.

If you find yourself spending most of your days indoors, you can do two things to keep your spirits up and your hormones pumping. First, install a "full-spectrum light" in your workplace. This light, produced by several companies in fluorescent tubes, emits the full spectrum of natural light waves from UV to infrared. Or you can get a plant grow-light (also full-spectrum) and install it to shine down on you while you work. You may not sprout, but at least you won't wither on the vine either.

Personality and Cancer

A personality is not something we emerge with fully formed at birth. We start out only with distinct leanings upon which we build a set of characteristic reactions and habits that taken together can be called our personality. We have more leeway than most of us think in choosing whether we will play up or play down those personality leanings. And it is possible to make changes if we find that some of those tendencies are damaging our health.

Recent research has uncovered certain distinct personality characteristics that do seem to be tied not only to the onset of cancer but to recovery as well.

Fighters—people who can express rather than repress anger and emotions—generally seem to have less chance of developing cancer and a greater chance of surviving it. This does not mean they are angry or highly emotional—as discussed in chapter 6, "Heart Disease," that would certainly not be healthy either. But they are comfortable about feeling and sharing with others the normal range of emotions.

Cancer patients tend to be low-intensity people who do not express their internal feelings easily and are not as close to their parents as those who develop hypertension, heart disease, or no serious disorder at all, according to a Johns Hopkins University researcher who has been studying 1337 men and women, most graduates from medical school classes from 1948–64, to see what factors lead to various diseases.

Those who feel depressed often, especially those experiencing a sense of hopelessness as a dominant part of their personality, seem to be highly at risk for developing cancer. One researcher interviewed a group of women all of whom showed suspicious cell changes in the cervix that had not yet been conclusively diagnosed as cancerous. The University of Rochester researcher did not look at their lab results, he simply gave them a personality test to measure "hopelessness." He predicted which would eventually get cancer based solely on their personalities—and he predicted with 70 percent accuracy.

Among a group of women (under study at Johns Hopkins University School of Medicine) who received drug treatment for spreading breast cancer, those who died earliest tended to suppress or deny their anger about their illness; those who survived the longest (over twenty-two months) were able to express their anger toward their condition and the doctor.

The theory here, as in all links of personality and disease, is that how you feel affects everything, including your immune system's ability to fight off cancer. There is still debate over which comes first—the mood or the disease. Cancer cells produce hormones themselves which might change psychological characteristics before the disease is detected.

But those who believe that attitude and personality are influencing the course of disease argue that fighting makes us feel as if we're still in control. And as we now understand with the stress response, the root of the negative effects of stress lies in that same feeling of helplessness and hopelessness—of having lost control of one's health, one's life. When that occurs, the immune system becomes depressed, and our vulnerability increases.

Some researchers believe that restoring that feeling of being in control of one's illness can repair the ravages of disease by energizing the immune system. Carl Simonton, a radiation oncologist and his wife, Stephanie, a psychologist, were two of the first to test this notion. At their Cancer Counseling and Research Center in Fort Worth, Texas, they combine standard medical therapy with a program that teaches cancer patients to visualize their immune system's white blood cells attacking and defeating the cancer cells (just as the little boy with brain cancer, discussed in chapter 2, did at the Menninger Clinic). The Simontons report—and they are getting some attention from more conservative members of the medical community—that of 159 patients who were diagnosed as being "medically incurable" with at most a year to live, the average survival time for those who died was 20.3 months. And of the 63 who survived, 22.2 percent show "no evidence of the disease."

The Simontons believe that visualization therapy—mobilizing the confidence of the individual to activate his or her immune system—can also be useful as a preventive measure for cancer and other serious ailments as well.

Until very recently, some would have scorned visualization therapy as quackery. Now it is being seriously considered as adjunct treatment by many respected researchers. It has become an integral part of athletic training for Olympic and professional athletes from international skiers (Jean-Claude Killy) to golf pros (Jack Nicklaus) and weight lifters (Arnold Schwarzenegger). Visualization can actually rehearse muscular coordination as effectively as actual physical rehearsal, and thus can enhance training. The technique is also being used to aid relaxation.

Some still say visualization achieves "only" the placebo effect. But the link between the mind and body, the placebo effect, is hardly hokum. It is evidence of our ability to activate healing processes within. It is a continuation of that great American tradition of pulling yourself up by your own bootstraps: it is you telling yourself to live, to get healthy, and for once in your life you are paying attention.

CANCER SUMMARY: RISKS, SYMPTOMS, PREVENTION

LUNG CANCER

INCIDENCE:
135,000 new cases this year

WHO DIES:
117,000 deaths a year

RISK FACTORS:
Cigarette smoking—those smoking 2 or more packs a day have death rates 15 to 25 times greater than nonsmokers
Exposure to industrial substances such as asbestos, nickel, chromates, or radioactive material, especially if you smoke
A history of tuberculosis

WARNING SIGNS:
Persistent cough
Sputum streaked with blood
Chest pain lasting more than a month
Chest colds more than three times a year
Recurrent attacks of pneumonia or bronchitis

TESTS TO DETECT EARLY:
Chest X ray
Sputum cytology
Fiberoptic bronchoscopy

PREVENTION TIPS:
Quit smoking or at least cut back—risk is proportional to the amount smoked
If you must smoke, do so only in well-ventilated areas so as not to compound the dangers by inhaling secondary smoke as well
Eat plenty of fruits and vegetables rich in vitamins C and A
Avoid exposure to irritating fumes—wear a mask if you must encounter them at work or at home while painting or spraying in the garden
Exercise regularly to strengthen lungs

COLON AND RECTUM CANCER

INCIDENCE:
126,000 new cases this year

WHO DIES:
58,000 deaths a year

RISK FACTORS:
Family history of the disease
Family history of polyps in the colon or rectum
Ulcerative colitis

WARNING SIGNS:
Bleeding from the rectum
Blood in the stool
Change in bowel habits

TESTS TO DETECT EARLY:
Digital rectal examination annually after age 40
Stool guaiac slide test, which can be done at home, yearly after age 50
Proctosigmoidoscopy (called a "procto") is recommended every 3 to 5 years after age 50 (after you have had 2 negative tests in consecutive years)

PREVENTION TIPS:
Avoid fatty meat in favor of chicken and fish
Reduce all fats and cholesterol in the diet
Eat more fruits and vegetables and whole grains for their fiber content as well as for vitamins A and C
Use alcohol only in moderation
Exercise—it helps avoid constipation

BREAST CANCER

INCIDENCE:
115,000 new cases this year; about 1 in 11 women get it

WHO DIES:
37,000 deaths a year

RISK FACTORS:
Family history of breast cancer before menopause
Never have had children
First child after age 30
Over age 35 and have had cancer in one breast
All women over age 50

WARNING SIGNS:
Changes in the breast size or shape
Swelling
Dimpling
Retraction of the nipple
Bloody or unusual discharge at the nipple
Scaliness or skin irritation
Pain or tenderness
A firm lump

TESTS TO DETECT EARLY:
Monthly breast self-exam for women over 20 (see end of chapter for instructions on a new, more sensitive exam technique)
Professional breast exam yearly—insist the gynecologist take adequate time
Ultrasound can determine if a lump is merely a cyst
X-ray mammography biennially for those over 40 or at high risk, annually for those over 50 or at high risk

PREVENTION TIPS:
Eat less fat, primarily by cutting back on red meat in favor of chicken and fish
Increase the fruits, vegetables, and whole grains in the diet, especially those rich in vitamin A
Consume alcohol only in moderation
Cut back on caffeine if you are at high risk

PROSTATE CANCER

INCIDENCE:
75,000 cases this year

WHO DIES:
24,000 a year

RISK FACTORS:
History of venereal disease
Diets high in fats, both saturated and unsaturated
Family history of prostate cancer increases risk slightly
Over age 50, risk increases

WARNING SIGNS:
Difficulty starting or stopping urine flow
Painful urination
Need to urinate frequently at night
Blood in the urine
Continuing pain in lower back, pelvis, or upper thighs
An irregular or unusually firm area in the prostate

TESTS TO DETECT EARLY:
Regular rectal exam after 40

PREVENTION TIPS:
Cut back on fat consumption
Eat fruits high in vitamin C
Eat vegetables rich in vitamin A as well as fiber

UTERINE CANCER

INCIDENCE:
55,000 new cases this year (16,000 of the cervix, 39,000 of the endometrium)

WHO DIES:
7000 deaths a year, 3000 from endometrial

RISK FACTORS:
Cervical cancer—Early age of first intercourse; Many sex partners; Genital herpes
Endometrial cancer—History of infertility; Failure to ovulate; Prolonged estrogen therapy; Late menopause; Diabetes, high blood pressure, and obesity

WARNING SIGNS:
Unusual bleeding or discharge

TESTS TO DETECT EARLY:
Pap test (which is very effective at detecting cervical but only 50 percent effective in detecting endometrial cancer) is advisable yearly for two years, then if both results were negative, you can take it every three years. If high risk, take it yearly.
Those at high risk of endometrial cancer should have an endometrial tissue sample at menopause
Pelvic exam by gynecologist at least every three years until age 40, annually after that

PREVENTION TIPS:
Lose weight if you are overweight
Eat less saturated and polyunsaturated fat—cancers of the ovary and endometrium may be linked to high blood levels of cholesterol and fatty diets
Eat more fruits rich in vitamin C—the equivalent of a couple of oranges a day
Increase folic acid in the diet—foods such as kidney, liver, yeast, and green vegetables

Reduce salt intake if you have high blood pressure
Avoid the use of talcum powder in the vaginal area—talc works its way
into internal organs, may cause ovarian cancer, and could affect these
cancers of the reproductive organs as well

ORAL CANCER

INCIDENCE:
27,000 new cases this year

WHO DIES:
9200 deaths a year

RISK FACTORS:
Heavy smoking
Heavy drinking
Use of chewing tobacco
Ill-fitting dentures

WARNING SIGNS:
Sore that bleeds easily and doesn't heal
A lump or thickening
Reddish or whitish patch that persists
Difficulty in chewing, swallowing, or moving the jaws or tongue

TESTS TO DETECT EARLY:
Regular dental checkups

PREVENTION TIPS:
Avoid tobacco in all forms including chewing tobacco
Consume only modest amounts of alcohol—both alcohol and smoke
irritate the lips, tongue, mouth, and throat
Get dentures adjusted to avoid irritating the gums
Eliminate nervous habits (such as biting the lip or inside of the cheek)
that can irritate the lining of the mouth
Eat more fruits high in vitamin C

SKIN CANCER

INCIDENCE:
17,000 cases of malignant melanoma; 400,000 new cases of highly cur-
able basal or squamous-cell cancers

WHO DIES:
7100 deaths a year

RISK FACTORS:
Prolonged exposure to the sun—four hours a day, four months a year
Very fair complexion
Moles on soles of feet or areas chronically irritated by shaving or tight
clothing
Occupational exposure to coal tar, pitch, creosote, arsenic compounds,
and radium
Scars from severe burns

WARNING SIGNS:

Any change in skin condition, especially the appearance of new moles—back, legs, and arms are common sites

Changes in the size or color of existing mole or other darkly pigmented spot

Look for the red, white, and blue syndrome—white spots within a pigmented area or with a reddish ring around it or the pigmented area turning a bluish color

A pale waxlike, pearly nodule cropping up

Or a red, scaly, sharply outlined patch

Bleeding from a mole

Irregular elevations on the surface of a mole

PREVENTION TIPS:

Avoid the sun from 10:00 A.M. to 3:00 P.M. when the ultraviolet rays are strongest

Wear protective clothing when you must be in the sun—darker colors keep out more light than light-colored clothing

Use sun screens with ingredients such as PABA

Consider moving if you are seriously at risk and live in California, Florida, or other area with a latitude near the equator

Avoid contact with arsenic (found in some insecticides) and coal-tar derivatives

Eat more vegetables and milk products rich in vitamin A

Avoid tight clothing that can irritate the skin

Caution: Seven General Warning Signs of Cancer*

C   Change in bladder or bowel habits.
A   A sore that does not heal.
U   Unusual bleeding or discharge.
T   Thickening or lump in breast or elsewhere.
I   Indigestion or difficulty in swallowing.
O   Obvious change in wart or mole.
N   Nagging cough or hoarseness.

Breast Self-Exam—A New and Thorough Technique

You've heard the advice a thousand times—*check your breasts.* I know it, you know it, we all know it, and none of us wants to do it. You've heard the excuses, too. "I forget what point in my monthly cycle I'm supposed to do it"; "I can't remember all the positions you're supposed to get into"; "Lord, with all these ridges and squidgy lumps

*From the American Cancer Society.

in there, how am I supposed to know what's normal or not?"

It seems more nerve-racking to check yourself than not to bother, right?

Wrong.

Do it.

Breast cancer is the most common cancer among women, touching one out of eleven women at some point in their lives, and taking the lives of 37,000 women a year. But lives can be saved if you catch the symptoms early enough. Nine out of ten women who are treated early for breast cancer are still alive five years later. Eighty percent of the lumps women find are benign. Stop worrying, start feeling.

Here is a new approach—a refinement of the old approach—that will enable you to detect even the smallest lumps. Be patient. If you are not used to examining yourself, you will be confused about what you feel. It takes time to get to know your body, but with regular examination, your breasts will become more familiar terrain than the back of your hand. And you will be equipped far better than most physicians to detect any slight change in your breast before serious trouble begins. Here's how to do it.

Look

Begin simply by looking. Stand in front of a mirror—first with arms at your side and then with arms raised above the head, and then with hands on your hips—to see if you notice any changes in your breasts. (For most women, one breast is larger than the other.) Look for:

- Any change in the shape of the breasts.
- Sore or swollen breasts, and pain or a lump or swelling under or around the arm.
- Inverted nipple.
- Rash on the breast, itching or dimpling of the breast.
- Hardness or indentation on the breast.
- Bloody or suspicious discharge from the nipple.

Feel: Think in Threes

Now the feeling begins. You can do a cursory exam anywhere, in the shower or in the bath. But for the most thorough job, you should lie on your back in a comfortable spot—the bed or a pad on the floor.

To examine the right breast, lie on your back but lean slightly to the left so the breast settles its weight evenly and doesn't pull to the right as it will (especially if you have large breasts) when you are flat on your back. Use pillows to prop you up comfortably. Lift your right arm up and rest the back of your hand on your forehead (or wherever it is comfortable and does not tense the chest muscle).

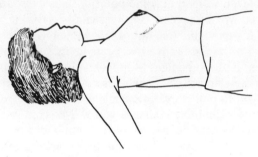

The examination proceeds in threes—three fingers do three circular rotations at three different levels of pressure for each spot on the breast.

Use your first three fingers—not just two—to do the feeling. Hold them out straight, though not stiffly, as you move around the breast so that the pads of the fingers—not the fingertips—do the exploring. The pads have proved to be far more sensitive (sensitive enough to read tiny Braille letters) than the tips in finding lumps.*

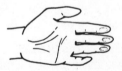

At each point on the breast your fingers will make three small circles about the size of a dime. With the first circle you should use light pressure, just feeling the surface of the skin. With the second circle you should press midway into the breast. And with the third circle you should press as deeply as you can go without causing discomfort. Lumps can exist at all levels, and using too little or too much pressure can make you miss one.

---

*The researchers at the University of Florida who developed the more sensitive system of breast examination upon which the advice here is based have formed Mammatech Corporation, which sponsors centers around the country to teach this new approach. Participants also get to feel a silicone breast with simulated lumps of all consistencies and at various depths in the "breast tissue" so that they can get a very clear sense of what to look for when examining themselves.

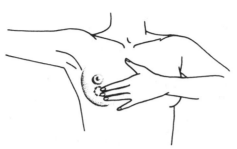

What Area to Cover

The breast area that must be examined extends much farther than the part of the breast that protrudes. Lumps can be found as high up as your collarbone or shoulder bone, into the armpit, and an inch below the breast.

To cover this whole area thoroughly without missing a spot, it helps to think of the breast area as a grid, composed of thin parallel lines much like the ribbed rows on a hand-knitted sweater.

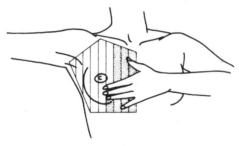

Begin at the top of the armpit and move slowly downward, making circles in threes without missing any space between the circles.

When you get to the bottom of the line, use the finger of the hand not doing the examining to mark your spot, then place your examining fingers just inside of that marker finger—in short, a finger width in—and continue in a straight line back upward. When you get to the top, mark your spot again, and then proceed with your circles down the next line.

Thinking of the breast area as a grid like this helps you examine much more thoroughly than the old approach taught in most books of simply circling the breast haphazardly or thinking of the breast as being divided into four quadrants.

Go very slowly, especially at first when you are getting the hang of it. It will take about ten minutes for each breast at first, so be patient.

Lumps

What does a lump really feel like?

Women ask this question because in the beginning, when you start feeling your own breasts, you notice what you think are lots of lumps. After a while you will get used to these soft, fibrous nodules—they used to be referred to as fibroid disease but are now regarded as perfectly normal breast tissue. And you will readily be able to tell the difference between fibrous tissue and a suspicious lump.

A lump can take many forms, but it usually is small and fairly hard. It can feel like a sharp pebble, an olive pit, a marble, or a bit softer like a firm, tiny rubber ball. It can stay in place or move around slightly; it can be right beneath the skin or way down deep in the breast. If it is something other than a normal fibrous lump, there will not be a symmetrical matching lump on the other breast.

Most lumps are benign. But all lumps should be examined by a doctor.

When to Do It

The best time to do the exam is three to seven days after your period, when the breasts are least likely to be sore or swollen. If you don't menstruate, pick any time—say, the day of the month your birthday falls on, so you'll remember it—and repeat it at the same time each month.

Who's at High Risk?

If close relatives, including a mother, sister, aunt or niece, has had breast cancer *before menopause,* then your chances may be two to three times higher than normal of also contracting it. If the cancer was in both breasts, your risk becomes higher still. However, if the breast cancer occurred after menopause, your chances are not affected one way or the other.

The younger you are when you bear your first child, the lower your risk. But the number of children you deliver has no bearing on your chances nor does breast-feeding protect you.

Those who have taken the birth control pill, contrary to earlier negative reports, may actually have better chances for recovery if they have already contracted breast cancer than those who have not taken the pill.

A small percentage of the more than half of all women who have a benign condition known as fibrocystic disease (which gives the breasts a lumpy feeling) may have a higher chance of developing breast cancer, but there is still no conclusive evidence.

And those who eat diets high in fat and low in fiber are putting themselves at risk.

For those at high risk, mammography (a breast X ray) may be advisable periodically. Those over age 50 (according to the National Cancer Institute) and over 40 (according to the American Cancer Society) should have annual mammograms. Technical advances have cut back the radiation from mammography X rays to anywhere from one-half to one-tenth the levels a few years ago, if new machinery and techniques are used. Shop around until you find a facility with up-to-date machinery; the two views of each breast involved in a standard mammography should deliver no more than one rad of radiation to the midbreast.

8
Diabetes and Arthritis

DIABETES

DIABETES IS ON THE RISE. It affects about 10 million Americans now, and the rate is growing 6 percent a year as Americans get older, fatter, and less active. Diabetes, one of the top-ten causes of death, not only kills 300,000 a year but also makes a sufferer more vulnerable to heart attacks, stroke, kidney failure, and blindness. Five million people may have the disease without knowing it.

That's the bad news.

The good news is that there is a growing understanding of what causes the disorder and a realization that for many diabetics—perhaps 60 to 70 percent, according to the American Diabetic Association—programs of diet and exercise and stress management may work better than drugs to cure it. Diabetes can be controlled, and diabetics can live normal, healthy lives.

Diabetes is a hormonal problem rendering the body unable to handle sugar adequately—the nutritional source for every cell in the body. Normally, the hormone insulin takes sugar from the bloodstream into the body's cells. But for diabetics—whether they haven't enough insulin or their bodies aren't paying attention to the insulin there—sugar builds up in the bloodstream and eventually damages blood vessels. In addition to suffering the complications of vascular damage (from gangrene in the feet, where blood vessels are narrow, to heart disease), diabetics also run the risk of falling into a diabetic coma because of blood-sugar imbalance.

Doctors have only recently come to recognize that many diabetics are not so much deficient in insulin as they are resistant to making use of the insulin their bodies do produce. The majority of diabetics who develop diabetes after age forty (late-onset diabetes) usually produce adequate amounts of insulin but their bodies ignore it and thus do not burn and store sugars properly. Only 5 percent of diabetics experience the disease from childhood, when it is an indication that the pancreas is not producing insulin.

How can we make the body use the existing insulin and avoid the need for artificial supplies? One answer can be found in life-style. Being overweight and underexercised diminishes and desensitizes the body cells' receptors for insulin. It is no coincidence that these are two conditions that affect a large number of diabetics. Experiencing stress can also raise blood-sugar levels.

In short, learning to control weight, exercise, and reactions under stress can go a long way toward bringing blood-sugar levels back to normal and reducing—often even eliminating—the diabetic's need for injected insulin or oral doses of hypoglycemic drugs. Even for those who do need insulin and other drugs and will for the rest of their lives, making modifications in diet, exercise, and stress reduction can lower the doses of drugs they need and improve their condition and their feelings of good health.

What to Do

If you notice some of the symptoms of diabetes (see the summary of symptoms later in this chapter), see a doctor and explain that you want to take an active role in your own care. Once diagnosed, a diabetic condition must be constantly monitored, but that does not mean that you will spend your life feeling sick. Especially if you follow these simple steps.

1. Lose weight.

   Whether being overweight can actually bring on diabetes or simply aggravate it in those already predisposed no one can say. But one thing is known: diabetics are more overweight than average. And simply losing weight can often immediately reduce or eliminate the need for insulin and other medicines.
2. Make sure your diet is high in fiber and whole-grain carbohydrates and low in refined sugar, fats, and modest in overall calories.

   A diet composed largely of fish, chicken, fruits, vegetables, and skim milk is the best bet, both to lose weight and to stay at your desired weight. Learning not only what to eat but when throughout the day, according to your own needs, can help keep your blood sugar level balanced.

3. Exercise regularly.

In addition to helping you lose weight and feel cheerful and healthy, physical activity uses sugar in the blood and seems to improve the body's sensitivity to insulin.

A good diet and exercise regimen, in addition to easing the diabetes, also reduces cholesterol and thus lowers the risk of hardening of the arteries that diabetics are especially sensitive to. Diabetics have two to four times the normal incidence of heart attacks and a higher incidence of strokes as well.

Doctors who have prescribed exercise and diet regimens—even for patients who were on as much as twenty to thirty units of insulin daily—report that they often can take patients off insulin entirely. But you must get professional advice on any new exercise routine, as there are dangers in lowering blood-sugar levels too quickly.

4. Stress reduction can improve your condition.

When under stress, your need for insulin rises. The hormones released under stress raise blood sugar levels. So a reduction in stress can be an important aid for diabetics (see chapter 12, "Learning to Love Stress," for a rundown on stress-control techniques).

However, there could be some problems in trying relaxation therapy on your own, if you're not adequately prepared. You may be so effective that your blood sugar levels drop too quickly and can bring about an insulin or hypoglycemic reaction. You may also need lower dosages of drugs as you master relaxation. Get advice from a doctor on how to proceed. As with vigorous exercise, it may be necessary to take a little extra mouthful of a carbohydrate before you begin.

If after vigorous exercise or trying stress reduction you experience weakness, hunger, sweating, faintness, shakiness, nervousness, or mental confusion, stop what you are doing. These are symptoms of dropping blood sugar levels. You may need to drink sugar water or fruit juice or inject an ampule of glucagon if your doctor has prescribed it.

5. Take special care of your feet.

Diabetes can cause hardening of the small arteries in the feet, which reduces resistance to infections and reduces sensation. The combination of those two factors means you can develop an infected toenail or callus without knowing it.

So you must inspect your feet daily. Bathe them often to keep them clean, be careful about cutting toenails, and attend to any calluses or irritations.

6. Be on the lookout for eye trouble.

Diabetes is the leading cause of blindness in adults aged twenty to sixty-five. But if you check out any changes in your vision, you should be able to prevent or reduce any loss of sight. There are new techniques (including a laser process) that are proving effective at halting complications. Be checked by a specialist, as many physicians do not know how to diagnose diabetic eye disease.

7. Even for those dependent on insulin, following the diet, exercise, stress reduction, and other self-help procedures can bring about significant improvements in your condition.

Self-help training programs are cropping up across the country to teach diabetics to monitor their blood sugar levels throughout the day (with blood and urine tests) and to keep them in the normal range through a judicious combination of drugs, exercise, controlled diet, and stress reduction.

8. If, after eating too much sugar or not eating enough food, the blood sugar levels swing dramatically high or low, there is the risk of entering a diabetic coma or going into insulin shock. For the symptoms and treatment of both, turn to chapter 17, "Self-Help Medical Aid."

Diabetes Summary

INCIDENCE

Ten million have diabetes; 300,000 die each year from it and its complications.

EARLY WARNING SIGNS

- Bruises and cuts may heal more slowly than usual.
- Skin itches or becomes infected more often than usual.
- You feel thirsty and hungry a great deal.
- You need to urinate more often than usual—possibly every hour.
- You feel tired.
- You lose weight without changing eating habits.
- Your vision changes.

EARLY DETECTION

It can be detected with simple urine and blood tests, which should be taken routinely every few years, especially after age forty. Your risk increases after age forty, especially if you have a family history of the disease (though even if both parents are diabetic, you have only a 1 in 20 risk of developing the insulin-dependent variety).

PREVENTION TIPS
1. Achieve and maintain your ideal body weight.
2. Eat a healthy diet, high in fiber and low in refined sugars, saturated fats, and cholesterol.
3. Exercise regularly.
4. Master stress-reduction techniques.

ARTHRITIS

The picture on this disease is finally looking better. Until very recently the prevailing medical opinion was that arthritis (osteoarthritis, that is) was just one of those diseases that was inevitable in old age. After all, dinosaurs had it, and the bones of Neanderthal man and Egyptian mummies have been found to show signs too.

But now, mummies or no, medical opinion is challenging the notion that there is nothing we can do in the face of arthritis. Most of us who live past 60 will show some signs of osteoarthritic wear and tear, but for many of us those signs will be insignificant, showing up only on X rays, not as aches and pains in our daily lives. If we pay attention to our weight, exercise, and stress-reduction procedures, we can go a long way in preventing and reducing arthritic symptoms and complications.

Arthritis does not usually kill but it does bring more pain and disability than it needs to. People spend nearly as many days in bed suffering from arthritis as from heart disease. Arthritis can be more than a pain in the neck, but there is also much we can do to make it less.

What Is Arthritis?

Of the hundred varieties of rheumatic diseases that have been identified, there are two kinds of arthritis that afflict the greatest number of people: osteoarthritis, more common as we age, and rheumatoid arthritis, which is rarer and more severe and affects not just a few joints but the whole body and internal organs as well.

OSTEOARTHRITIS

Osteoarthritis touches about 40 million men and women, mostly over age fifty. The problem arises when the cartilage, the tough elastic substance that covers the ends of bones where they meet within a joint, is worn down and no longer adequately cushions and protects the bones as we move.

The question that cannot be fully answered is why the cartilage wears down. Obviously, cartilage suffers some wear and tear just from our living and aging. But there is a reason some people experience arthritic problems earlier and more severely than others. And while genetic predisposition may certainly play a part, it is even more certain that many things we do to ourselves can make us more or less likely to suffer from this disease.

Excessive weight, chronic bad posture, habitual tensing of muscles under stress, and occupational overuse or injury of a specific joint repeatedly (baseball pitchers and ballet dancers are the most glamorous examples) can all put more strain on joints than they can tolerate. They can bring on the disease or aggravate an existing condition, and changing some of those conditions and habits can also eliminate or alleviate the pain and stiffness the disorder brings.

RHEUMATOID ARTHRITIS

Rheumatoid arthritis, the most difficult to control and severely damaging of the rheumatic diseases, affects 6.5 million people. It can strike anytime, usually between ages twenty and forty-five, and affects three times as many women as men. Juvenile rheumatoid arthritis, hitting children from infancy to their teens, at the present time affects about 250,000. (Two-thirds of the children who get it will recover by adulthood.)

With this disease, you can experience red, hot, inflamed joints in a few spots or all over the body. The damage may spread to organs such as the heart, lungs, spleen, nerves, and eyes. Usually the first areas hit are the small joints in the hands and the heavy weight-bearing joints of the knees, hips, neck, and spine. Tissues lining the joints become inflamed and thicken, causing pain and swelling and eventually—if no action is taken—may actually destroy the cartilage and bone and result in deformity.

No one knows exactly what causes this disorder. It could be a virus that triggers the inflammation. In any event, what happens next seems to be that the immune system goes out of whack in responding to the inflammation. The body (in what is termed an autoimmune response, as occurs in allergic reactions) begins a kind of war against itself, and the joints are the war zone.

With rheumatoid arthritis as well as osteoarthritis, emotional stress seems to speed up progress of the disease and make it worse. When stress is relieved, the condition seems to improve. Being overweight also adds considerably to the strain on the joints, as does poor posture and lack of exercise.

GOUT, BURSITIS, TENDONITIS

Gout, reputed to be the disease of the overindulgent rich, is actually another form of arthritis affecting 1.6 million Americans, mostly men. It commonly strikes a foot joint, usually the big toe. Uric acid crystals build up in the joints, causing inflammation and pain.

The link of gout to overindulgence is not totally off the mark. It is the one form of arthritis in which food unquestionably plays a part in triggering and curing the disease.

Purine-rich foods—anchovies, organ meats, scallops, peas, and beans—as well as alcohol consumption can trigger bouts of gout. And abstention from both rich food and drink can bring decided improvement.

Bursitis and tendonitis, while less serious, can still be painful. These ailments affect structures surrounding the joints, an inflammation usually arising from a specific injury or repeated strain. "Housemaid's knee" and "tennis elbow" or "tennis shoulder" (which you can get from other activities as well) are the most common examples.

What You Can Do to Prevent and Treat Arthritis

The general prevention tactics are much the same for rheumatoid arthritis and osteoarthritis.

The first step, if you notice any of the symptoms listed below, is to see a doctor. Delaying can mean you are allowing joint damage to proceed when you could be stopping it. Beware of magic cures. Quackery abounds in the treatment of arthritis. For every $1 spent on legitimate arthritis research, sufferers spend $25 on phony "cures," including everything from alfalfa, seawater, and yucca tablets to copper bracelets, salves, and "wonder" drugs that are simply aspirin in expensive disguise.

1. Exercise daily.

    Routine exercise builds strong ligaments and tendons which support the joints and keep cartilage healthy. If you don't exercise, joints stiffen, cartilage deteriorates, and muscles start to atrophy. Exercise also slows down the demineralization of bones that comes with age and makes us more vulnerable to arthritic wear.

    The best exercises are those that stimulate joints, rotating them through the full range of motion without jarring them—swimming or brisk walking head the list. If you are already in good shape, dance, tennis, running, handball, and soccer can be good sports as well. Working out at least fifteen minutes every day is probably the best schedule.

2. Pick an exercise that is vigorous but does not place particular strain on any one joint.

    Baseball pitching, even if you cannot get the ball over the plate at 90 miles per hour the way the pros do, can still prove more strain than stimulation. Baseball pitchers often develop osteoarthritis early in life in their pitching arms because of this unnatural and difficult movement.

    Ballet dancers, too, are more prone than others to get osteoarthritis in their ankles, again because of the strain that the unnatural toe-stand places on those joints. But bear in mind that professionals, who work vigorously on their movement six to eight hours a day for years, are in more precarious positions than those of us who pick dance or a sport as exercise three to five times a week. So don't be too cautious in your selection.

3. Learn proper posture to ease pressure on the joints.

    Incorrect posture can encourage deformities and contractures in joints and aggravate neck, back, shoulder, and even hip pain. Many of us may not really know what good posture is and may be doing ourselves damage unwittingly.

4. Rest painful parts, but don't let pain immobilize you.

    Short periods of rest are necessary to allow an already sore joint to recover. But don't dawdle about getting moving again. If you allow pain in one joint to limit or alter movement, you can set off a chain reaction, making pain and stiffness spread well beyond the initial offending joint. For example, if one hip hurts, and you start favoring it, you will be distorting the body alignment, twisting the spine and a host of muscles, putting excessive strain on the other joint, and eventually spreading trouble. The underused joint can grow so stiff that it can actually lock into place, eventually preventing you from standing or lying straight.

5. Use aspirin to reduce pain, stiffness, and inflammation.

Aspirin is still the safest and most effective drug available for arthritis. It reduces pain enough to encourage you to move and stimulate the joints naturally.

Aspirin is also therapeutic. For those with rheumatoid arthritis, it can effectively reduce inflammation, thereby preventing further damage to tissue and cartilage. The only problem is that aspirin must be taken in high doses, perhaps twenty pills a day, every day, whether or not you are in pain, to be effective. To prevent the digestive upsets that aspirin can cause, take it at mealtimes, with food and lots of water, and take the enteric-coated variety that doesn't dissolve in the stomach but waits until it gets to the intestines. Buffered aspirin, taken at these high doses, does not provide any greater protection than the ordinary aspirin.

There are other antiarthritis drugs given by prescription if aspirin does not prove effective. Consult a physician and discuss the side effects.

6. Maintain a normal body weight—diet if you are overweight.

People more than 10 percent over their ideal weight have twice the incidence of osteoarthritis. Every extra pound you carry around puts additional strain on your joints and adds pain to your movements. Wear shoes with good support for the ankle and rubber or crepe soles that absorb the shock that travels up the bones and joints as you walk.

7. Massage and moist heat help ease pain and encourage stimulating movement.

Massaging the muscles around the sore joint (rather than the joint itself) stimulates blood supply to the muscles and tissues around the joint and eases pain. Moist heat does the same. Soaking in a warm bath or shower is excellent for pain as well as relaxation. If you do it before exercising, it will loosen up muscles and joints and reduce chances of injury. If you do it afterward as well, you may be able to ward off that postworkout stiffness.

8. Sleep on a good, firm bed—sagging into a soft mattress puts strain on muscles and joints.

If arthritis has given you back pain, you should try sleeping on your side or your back (not on your stomach) on a very firm mattress. The pillow should be thin so that your head and neck stay in straight alignment with your spine. (A down pillow works best as it can be fluffed up and folded or flattened to the varying thicknesses necessary as you shift from back to side positions.)

9. Use stress-reduction techniques throughout the day as small tensions develop.

Reducing stress eases muscular tension that can lead to aches and pains and strains throughout the body. Many of the techniques you will find in chapter 12, "Learning to Love Stress," are useful not only for defusing stress but for reducing pain as well. The elements borrowed from hypnosis in the Ten-Second Stress Fix can help you control the aches and pain that flare up during the day and allow you to concentrate on carrying out your normal activities. The other relaxation techniques can help you get a good night's sleep, too.

10. Keep up an active sex life.

In addition to the pleasurable sensations, sexual activities also stimulate the release of adrenaline and cortisone, which act as natural painkillers. Some researchers have estimated that good sex can give arthritics four to six hours of relief. Sex does not have to be intercourse, nor does it have to be with a partner. Any stimulation should bring about the release of these pain-relieving hormones.

11. Beware of quackery.

Loading up on "acid" fruits and vegetables or cutting out the "nightshades"—tomatoes, eggplant, peppers—or swallowing supplements of vitamins C, A, and B complex as even doctors advocated in the 1930s, have not been shown to do anything more than a healthy, normal diet.

Injections of gold salts, which sound suspicious, are actually a medically accepted treatment for some, though the procedure is not without its side effects and therefore is reserved for severe cases of rheumatoid arthritis.

12. Is there an arthritis diet?

Not exactly. Diet does play a role in certain types of arthritis such as gout and scurvy. However, links between specific foods and the leading types of arthritis have not yet been demonstrated. That doesn't mean there may not be such a link, but it is too soon to say what it might be. Arthritis is a collagen disease and vitamin C is necessary for forming collagen fiber, but no controlled studies have been done on the effects of vitamin C. Calcium may play a part, as this mineral is critical for strong bones, and many Americans who think their diets are well-rounded actually do not get enough calcium.

Some believe rheumatoid arthritis is caused in many instances by common food allergies—corn, milk, wheat, or lamb are often thought to be the culprits. But, again, there is not yet proof. It certainly cannot hurt to try cutting out certain foods for several weeks at a time to see if they might be adversely affecting you. Do not expect many doctors to be sympathetic with such efforts. And do not focus all your energies on diet to the exclusion of the other remedies that are more likely to yield soothing results.

Arthritis Summary

INCIDENCE
- Osteoarthritis—16 million have painful symptoms; perhaps 40 million would show up with signs on X ray but do not have severe symptoms.
- Rheumatoid arthritis—6.5 million, twice as many women as men.

EARLY WARNING SIGNS
1. Pain or achiness as you experience with a cold or flu in a joint that may spread to a nearby part of the body.
2. Stiffness, especially in the morning; redness or swelling at the joints. For juveniles—high fever and skin rash.
3. Nodules forming under the skin.
4. Loss of mobility so that you can't perform the usual movements easily—wrists, knuckles, and ankles are commonly affected.
5. Unexplained weight loss, fever, fatigue, or weakness in combination with joint problems.

PREVENTION TIPS
1. Lose weight if you are at all overweight.
2. Exercise regularly, choosing an activity that stretches and tones without jolting the joints.
3. Use aspirin, moist heat, and massage to reduce pain and inflammation.
4. Rest a sore joint, but don't get too much rest.
5. Eat a healthy, balanced diet, being especially conscious of getting adequate supplies (in foods, not supplements) of vitamin C and calcium.
6. Maintain good posture.
7. Wear shoes with soles that absorb the shock that moving brings to joints.
8. Sleep on a firm, supportive mattress.

9
Accidents

THE FIRST THING human beings did to set themselves apart was to stand on two legs.

The second thing they did was to trip.

Injuries are as old as mankind, and for a long time we accepted them as just one of those uncontrollable unpleasantnesses that go with living. But that is not the case—many accidents don't "just happen." It is only within the last few years that scientists have put their skills to the task of analyzing this area. It's not as sexy and dramatic as saving a victm after an accident has already taken place. The findings are that we—not the Fates—often influence the occurrence of many mishaps that can and should be prevented.

And the 75 million accidents that occur annually in America are more than a trifle unpleasant. They are the leading cause of death for people under forty years of age. They cost us time—29 million days in the hospital—and money—$18 billion a year on motor vehicle accidents alone, or about 1 percent of the gross national product. Accidents erase more productive years of life than any disease.

LATEST YEARLY ACCIDENT REPORT

Motor vehicles	46,000 deaths 1.7 million disabling injuries
Falls	11,600 deaths 11 million injuries
Drownings	6200 deaths
Burns	5000 deaths 60,000 hospital admissions for injuries
Poisonings	4400 deaths a year; 400,000 children treated a year
Gunshot wounds	31,000 deaths—2000 accidental, 12,900 homicide, 16,000 suicide

What Can We Do to Prevent Accidents?

We do not have to pamper ourselves in order to protect ourselves. Preventing accidents does not mean never taking risks. It means we shouldn't take stupid risks. And we should know where the risks lie so we can choose when to dare the Fates, and when it doesn't seem worth it.

"I just didn't think" is the most common phrase that springs to one's lips after an accident. I just didn't think the other car was going to turn; I didn't think my little girl could climb up into that cabinet where I kept the drain cleaner; I never thought the fire in the frying pan would spread so fast. Now's the time to think, while you're sitting here safe and snug. Run through the following step-by-step checklists of action you can take—in your habits and around your home or office—to reduce your chances for danger. You can't be expected to do everything; that's why the suggestions aim at only the most significant contributing causes of accidents. The checklists make it easy finally to take the protective measures you already knew you should.

Cars

Motor vehicle accidents are the leading cause of accidental death, and the numbers are rising.

Our behavior at the wheel is important, and the checklist will focus on that. But it is not the only relevant factor. Car manufacturers' choices in design also can make the critical difference between slight and severe injury or even death. Many of those choices involve very little expense.

For example, a study found that if cars were made with simply one extra brake light on the midline of the car or behind the rear window, rear-end collisions could be cut in half. Airbags, too, which inflate in milliseconds of a head-on collision (and which during extensive testing have almost never misfired), could save perhaps 12,000 lives and hundreds of thousands of injuries a year.

This is not to say that car makers have done nothing. In 1966 they introduced laminated windshields which have saved thousands yearly from dangerous and disfiguring lacerations. Bumpers are better, but they and a number of other features could be better still.

However, until those changes come to pass, car safety is up to us.

1. Do not drink and drive—drinking strongly increases your chances of being involved in a fatal accident.

   In 45 percent of fatal car accidents, someone involved has been drinking alcohol. A healthy liver can get rid of only one drink per hour. As your blood alcohol level rises, your reaction time slows and your judgment grows foggy. Driving in a fog, whether of your making or nature's, is never safe.

2. Don't let teenagers drive without supervision.

   Young drivers—because they are impetuous as well as inexperienced—cause most of the accidents. Driver's education programs do not help, according to accident specialists at Johns Hopkins University in Baltimore. In fact, these researchers say such programs actually increase fatal crashes because they put more young people on the road.

3. Before you turn the key in the ignition, put your seat belt on.

   Contrary to popular belief, seat belts will not trap you inside the car and thereby increase your danger in an accident. The reverse is actually true—people who are thrown out of a car during an accident have twenty-five times higher risk of dying than those wearing seat belts. Half of all automobile deaths, nearly all traumatic dislocations of the hip (60 to 90 percent result from auto accidents), and an even greater share of more common injuries could be prevented if people used seat belts.

   As the driver, you should insist that all passengers wear seat belts, too, especially children.

4. Infants and children should sit in the backseat and use either seat belts or protective infant seats.

   The backseat is safer than the front in most accidents. Infants—who should not be allowed to leave the hospital in a car unless parents have a safe infant's car seat—should face backward if they must be placed in the front seat.

   Simply holding an infant in your arms is not adequate protection. In a 30-mile-per-hour collision, a 10-pound child can exert 300 pounds of force against a parent's grip. In short, no parent could hold on. And the child's fragile body and soft head will be thrown like a billiard ball against windows and doors with crushing force.

5. Drive as slowly as you can stand it without holding up traffic.

   During the oil crisis in the mid-seventies, when fewer people drove and those who did faced strictly enforced 55-mile-per-hour limits, the annual death toll fell sharply below 50,000 for the first time in decades. As the oil shortage eased, and lines at gas stations shrank, drivers stopped worrying about saving fuel and returned to higher speeds, and the death toll went right back up.

6. Have the car inspected regularly to make sure it is in safe operating condition.

   In addition, check by yourself to make sure that brakes, windshield wipers, turn signals, lights, horn, and exhaust systems are all working properly.

7. If you are angry, don't get into the car.

   Take a walk around the block. Driving requires concentrated energy, and when you are angry you neither concentrate adequately nor have enough residual tolerance for the annoying situations that inevitably arise in the course of even the smoothest rides.

8. If you've been taking medication—especially cold medication or sedatives or tranquilizers—the only car you should be in is one driven by someone else.

9. Avoid driving in bad weather.

   Sounds obvious, but most of us don't appreciate how dramatically even a gentle rain can increase the chances of a serious accident. If you must go out, leave much more time than usual to get to your destination so you aren't tempted to take any risky shortcuts.

10. Travel secondary roads instead of interstates and superhighways whenever possible.

    Highway driving is exceptionally dangerous for your body (not to mention your soul). The roads are so boring as to be mesmerizing, and you have to maintain constant vigilance just to stay awake. In addition, you are driving very fast, which leaves little room for error or delay in reactions.

    On any road, the place to be especially careful is around the exit and entrance ramps. That's where most of the accidents happen.

Falls

Falls are the leading cause of injuries around the home. Fourteen million people are hurt, 15,000 are killed, with a majority of the incidents occurring around stairs or in the kitchen.

STAIRS

1. Mark the top and bottom step on the stairway.

    Many people trip down stairs because they don't notice where the first one begins or the last one ends; it's easy in both directions to mistake the next to the last for the last. A colored strip of adhesive or some colorful marking can set off these steps.
2. Cover stairs with carpet where possible.

    If you forgot to put the markings on the top and bottom stairs, and you tumble, carpeting can take some of the sting off the slip. No shag carpet—heels can catch.
3. Install handrails on outdoor steps.

    Rain, sleet, and snow may not stop the mail carriers, but it can stop the rest of us rather abruptly and painfully on concrete steps. Even if there are only a couple of steps, put up something to grab onto.
4. Don't negotiate steps in your socks or stockings.

FLOORS

1. Spilled grease or melting ice cubes, especially on a slick linoleum kitchen floor or cement patio, create slippery patches.

    It's all very well for someone to say, "Wipe up spills instantly," but who would listen? If you're in the middle of cooking and chopping ingredients, there isn't always time.

    So the advice here is that you should at least drop a handy paper towel, dishcloth, potholder, *anything,* on top of the spill to alert everyone to avoid that spot.

    Clean up later.
2. Small scatter rugs should have a nonskid liner underneath.

    An under carpet not only keeps the rug and the family from slipping but it protects the rug as well from wear and tear.

WINDOWS

1. Window guards help prevent serious falls from windows.

    Children are at most risk of falling out of windows. In 1973, New York City began giving families in high-rise, high-risk, city housing free, easy-to-install window guards. Two years later, the number of deaths by falls had decreased 35 percent.
2. Open windows by pushing the top window down rather than lifting up the bottom window, if you have the option; install screens.

    Again, this makes it more difficult for children to climb up and fall out.

Poisonings

If you think children are at the greatest mortal risk in accidental poisonings, you would be in agreement with a majority of people, but you would also be wrong. Only 2 percent of poisoning deaths involve children under age five. But you would be right in your impression that children are still at risk. Some 400,000 every year get into dangerous substances and require treatment. For adults and children, these are the most easily preventable kinds of mishaps.

ADULTS

1. Never take medicine in the dark.

    Even if you wake up in the middle of the night with a splitting headache and you think you know exactly where to reach for the aspirin bottle, turn on the light, prop open an eyelid, and read the label. There is very little difference among the feel of medicine containers.

2. Don't mix drugs—even over-the-counter drugs—unless you've checked with an expert about dangerous interactions.

    Two drugs, each of which may be safe taken alone, when combined can cause trouble. Alcohol and nearly any drug do not mix happily; with tranquilizers or antihistamines or even some cold medicines containing codeine, the results can be fatal. Aspirin, too, should not be mixed with many drugs, especially anticoagulants, as dangerous internal bleeding may result.

3. Spend as little time as possible around automobile exhaust. It is responsible for a large number of gas and vapor poisonings.

    Don't sit in the car—especially if it is in the garage—while warming up the engine in winter; don't stand in the garage for long either.

    Even if you are outdoors, carbon monoxide fumes can be dangerous if you stand too close to the exhaust while, for example, scraping ice off the back and side windows. If you must get close, take frequent breaks to move far from the exhaust and breathe the fresh air before returning.

4. Wear a Medic-Alert bracelet if you have any allergies or diseases someone should know about in an emergency.

CHILDREN

1. If you have a child in the house, buy all medication with safety caps. You may curse this 1972 innovation when you have a headache and

can't open the aspirin bottle, but it has lowered deaths from swallowing pain and fever pills by 41 percent since then.

2. Do not transfer toxic substances to other containers, especially not to tempting vessels like soda bottles or coffee cans (which many people use to store opened insecticides or turpentine for cleaning paintbrushes).

3. Move household cleaners out from under the sink and up high in hard-to-reach cupboards.

4. Put safety locks on medicine cabinets and even those cabinets you thought were hard to reach. Children can be devilishly agile when their curiosity is piqued.

5. Don't keep medicine—even vitamins and especially iron pills—on the kitchen table; they can be toxic for children.

6. When the child is very young, get rid of poisonous house plants: arnica, calla lily, castor bean, daffodil, dieffenbachia, dumb cane, elephant's ear, hyacinth, mistletoe, narcissus, oleander, philodendron, poinsettia, rosemary pea.

7. If all the precautions fail and the child swallows something dangerous, grab the bottle or package the substance came in along with the child, and call your state poison control center—the number should be by the phone. The labels of many household cleaners and poisons specify what action to take if someone ingests the poison. But some are wrong so don't do anything until the poison center advises you.

Drowning

1. Public and private pools alike should have protective fencing to keep people out when a lifeguard is not around. Fencing can save lives. Honolulu, which has the perfect weather for swimming, now requires protective fencing around all public and private swimming pools. Brisbane, Australia, a comparable city in weather and the popularity of the water sport, has no such law and has a death rate from drowning three times that of Honolulu.

2. Familiarize yourself with resuscitation and first-aid techniques.

3. Don't drink and swim; don't even get into a hot tub. More than one-third of all adults who drown have high levels of alcohol in their blood.

Fire, Burns, Scalds

Some 4100 people die every year from household fires and well over a million are hurt or disfigured by burns or scalds. Cigarettes set off half of all house fires; alcohol is implicated in 70 percent of all burn injuries.

FIRE

1. Put up a smoke alarm even if your state is one of the few remaining that has not passed a law requiring them.
2. Check to make sure you've turned off all appliances, oven and stove burners and emptied all ashtrays before going to bed.

   If you've had a party, also check rugs and upholstery for any stray live ashes or cigarette butts. Smokers can be frighteningly irresponsible about the disposal of their ashes. And a couch cushion could smolder for some time before building into flames.
3. Don't smoke in or around the bed.

   All it takes is a hot ash to start fatal trouble in the bedroom. A live ash on a mattress tends to smolder silently—no crackling flames that might awaken you and give you a chance to flee—and give off poisonous fumes from which there is no escape.
4. If grease catches fire in the kitchen, clap a pan lid over the flame. Do not throw water on it or pour water into a flaming frying pan as this will only spread the fire.

   To prevent grease from splattering everywhere in the kitchen and running the risk that a spark or a flame from the stove will set the grease burning, use a metal mesh pan cover while frying—it allows the moisture to escape but catches most of the splatterings. (If you're really concerned about your health, you should do less frying and use less fat, anyway.)
5. Keep a fire extinguisher on every floor in the home, and don't wait for an emergency to read the instructions on how to uncap it.

   Aim at the source of the fire, not the flames, and move the extinguisher from side to side. Household fires must be put out quickly or they get out of hand. It isn't usually the flames that are the danger, but the poisonous fumes that burning housing materials give off. Eighty percent of fire deaths result from inhaling these noxious fumes.

   If you can't put the fire out quickly, get out of the house to avoid the fumes.

6. If you live in an apartment, don't use elevators in a fire.
    They can be deathtraps if they are stuck between floors or they stay at the floor with the fire.

BURNS AND SCALDS
1. Make sure your water heater has a delay in delivering hot water, the cause of most household scalds. Also set it so that it doesn't deliver hotter water than you really need.

    Residential hot-water heaters can be modified so as not to heat water above 130 degrees F—first-degree burns result after 30 seconds of exposure to water at this temperature. Where there are very young children or elderly individuals who might take even longer to escape from a shower or bath accident, the top temperature should be set even lower. (Manufacturers could save a great deal of pain and suffering if they designed hot-water heaters to make these accommodations.)
2. Don't leave children alone in the bathtub lest they fiddle with the hot-water tap.
3. In the kitchen, turn all panhandles so they don't extend out beyond the stove. This will not only prevent curious children from grabbing at them and emptying the hot contents on themselves, it keeps adults from walking by and knocking the pot over.

Choking

More adults die from getting food stuck in their throats than from firearm accidents; for children under age five, choking is the second greatest cause of accidental death. For everyone, if the object blocking the air supply is not dislodged within about four minutes, permanent brain damage begins and death is not far behind.

If you could peer down the throat, you'd see why choking is so common. The opening at the top of the trachea or windpipe lies right next to the opening of the esophagus that leads into the stomach. With every swallow, one opening is supposed to close as the other opens, and most of us execute this muscular syncopation successfully hundreds of times a day. But sometimes there's a slipup. Alcohol, especially, can dull the reaction time, and it is implicated in 70 percent of adult chokings.

Parents must try to keep small, rubbery items out of youngsters' hands. They are perfect for chewing on and the most dangerous for slipping down the throat and wedging firmly. Small balls, even foods such as hot dogs, are common culprits. Adults and children alike must heed the advice of their mothers—chew your food slowly.

In an emergency, you must administer the Heimlich maneuver (see chapter 17, "Self-Help Medical Aid," for instructions with a variation for small children).

Insect Stings

Insects may seem to be everywhere, but their dangers are not unavoidable. They have special spots where they are more likely to be than others, just as we do. Knowing their habits can help us prevent meeting up with them in unfavorable circumstances.

1. Don't go barefoot in the clover; bees and yellow jackets are quite fond of ground clover. Yellow jackets seek out fragrant blossoms and fruits.
2. If you know you have to be outside in an area with a lot of bees or stinging insects, avoid wearing perfumes or hair spray and keep as much of your body covered as possible.
3. While you may not be able to avoid an encounter with a lone bee, you should be on the lookout for nests, as multiple stings can be quite dangerous even if you are not allergic. Yellow jackets burrow in the ground to make their home. Honeybees seek out hollows in trees or caves. Hornet hives often hang from trees.

Back Injuries

Falls can send your back out of whack, but the fitter you are, the safer you are from these injuries. First, if you are in shape and your muscles are strong and supple, it is likely that your reflexes will be quick enough to right your body rapidly after a small misstep and prevent these inevitable small slips from becoming full-fledged falls.

Second, even if you do fall, if you are fit, your developed stomach and back muscles will lessen the chances for serious wrenching damage.

Most back injuries stem not so much from a specific accidental incident so much as routine misuse and disuse of muscles. Poor posture as we sit or stand and undeveloped stomach muscles are largely the problems. The best protection you can give yourself, once you've done your best to prevent falls and auto accidents, is to learn correct posture and carry out the back exercises that will strengthen your back when the inevitable slip occurs.

And when you lift anything heavier than a martini, bend your knees and activate your leg and stomach muscles before you lift and put any strain on your back.

Stress

People under emotional stress are accident-prone. The accident rate doubles among those recently separated or divorced.

Frustration is a factor—waiting in line, letting annoyance build, makes people more inclined to take rash action. Children whose families suffer great stress (marital troubles, the death or illness of a close relative) have been shown to suffer more accidents and illnesses than children of families under less stress.

In addition, those under stress are more likely to want to smoke or drink or take drugs in the hope of alleviating the stress. All those activities increase the risks of fire, car accidents, falls, and just about every kind of accident imaginable.

The best advice here, since we cannot avoid stress, is to learn how to cope with it.

Reducing the Risks —Big and Small

HERE YOU'LL FIND the latest research on painless programs that really work to help you change your habits—how you eat, sleep, respond to stress—changes that last not just for a day but for the rest of your long healthy life.

10
Exercise: Why Start, Where to Start, and How to Keep It Up

THE FIRST AND MOST PRESSING question here is *why bother?* Working up a sweat at sports is not universally held in high regard. Robert Maynard Hutchins, renowned academic innovator and president of the University of Chicago in the 1930s, is reported to have announced, upon eliminating intercollegiate football at that university, "Of course even I feel the impulse to exercise occasionally—but I lie down until it passes."

Hutchins' sentiments, whether apocryphal or not, are still shared by many. While in opinion polls half of all adults claim to exercise, the truth is closer to 35 percent, according to the U.S. Public Health Service. We're doing better than a decade or two ago, yes. But we're hardly up to the levels of rigorous physical activity that humans have engaged in over the thousands of years of human evolution, a vigorous level at which our cardiovascular and endocrine and metabolic systems actually function best.

Sadder still, we are losing ground where it counts the most—among our children. At a time when they are most resilient and receptive to learning new movements and forming good habits that could last a lifetime, only one-third of schoolchildren participate daily in physical education programs, and that percentage is going down.

Until very recently, the medical profession, too, tended toward blasé dismissal of the role of exercise in good health. Few researchers bothered to study its effects.

But that is changing. In the last few years, scientific studies have begun. Exercise science is rapidly emerging as an important and respectable field of study. And now the benefits of exercise are no longer simply speculation. An impressive array of data confirm that human beings were not meant to be sedentary beasts.

Exercise can do much more than burn calories. It can be of benefit to your heart, bones, and brain, can help fight infection, diabetes, arthritis, and back pain, can lift your spirits, help you sleep, and lengthen your life. No matter how old you are, and no matter what your current condition—even if you cannot move out of a chair—you can improve your fitness and feel better for it.

I. Benefits of Exercise—Getting Out More Than You Put In

PROTECTS AGAINST HEART ATTACKS

Exercise seems to provide protection against not only the slow buildup of clogged arteries that can lead to heart attacks but also "sudden death" from heart attacks, even though this kind of coronary event used to be considered more random. People who jogged, chopped wood, or played singles tennis were shown in a Seattle study to have lower risk from a sudden heart attack than those pursuing a more sedentary life.

Men who are already at risk for heart disease from smoking, high blood pressure, or high cholesterol levels are six times safer from heart attacks if they exercise than men with the same risky habits who do not exercise and have low "physical work capacity," according to an eight-year investigation at the University of Southern California School of Medicine.

Even people who exercise only on weekends have been found in a British study to have fewer heart attacks than those who never exercise. Any activity that burns about 300 calories a day—such as an hour's brisk walk or a half hour of cycling—markedly lowers your chances for a heart attack according to studies by a Stanford University researcher.

And those who do go on to have a heart attack will likely suffer a milder one if they have been exercising and keeping fit.

Aerobic Exercise Lowers Pulse Rate

After you have exercised vigorously and regularly for several weeks, it is not uncommon for your resting pulse rate to go down 20 beats.

Think about how much work that saves your heart. If it beats 20 fewer times per minute, that's 28,800 beats a day; 10.5 million throbs a year saved. Any heart would be grateful.

CUTS FAT LEVELS IN THE BLOOD

Moderate exercise can raise the levels of the "good" cholesterol—HDLs, the high-density lipoproteins that protect against atherosclerosis by removing fats from the blood—while lowering the levels of the "bad" cholesterol—the LDLs, low-density lipoproteins that promote fatty deposits in the arteries.

In a monkey study—human beings are not usually amenable to living out their lives in a controlled laboratory environment—investigators from Boston University Medical Center had monkeys walk 1.2 to 2.2 miles per hour, a good walking pace, for one hour three times a week. Not only did the exercising monkeys have higher HDL levels and lower LDL levels, they had larger hearts, wider coronary arteries, and smaller fatty deposits than the control monkeys.

So even moderate exercise may prevent or retard heart disease in primates, and man is king of the primates.

LOWERS BLOOD PRESSURE

Men who burn 2000 kilocalories per week (the equivalent of a strenuous aerobic workout four or five times a week) have been found to be 23 percent less likely to develop hypertension than their sedentary counterparts. In some cases, exercise eliminates any need for drugs in bringing high blood pressure down to normal.

Exercise, by reducing blood pressure and thus hypertension, ultimately wards off heart attacks and strokes.

PREVENTS ANGINA

An exercise training program can be as potent as nitroglycerin in alleviating or preventing angina.

Once you're fit and have increased your endurance, heart rate and blood pressure go down, enabling you to do more before you tax the oxygen supply and angina pain begins.

EUPHORIA—THE EXERCISE HIGH

Vigorous exercise—and it needn't be running, though the feeling has been called "runner's high"—can produce a euphoric or "high" feeling that works wonders in fighting depression. One California psychiatrist says he finds taking a weekly run with his depressed schizophrenic patients has proved more effective than conventional analysis and drug therapy.

No one knows exactly why this happens but it seems to be related to an increase, during exertion, in the body's levels of endorphins, chemicals much like morphine that the brain naturally produces. Morphine is an excellent painkiller and produces a euphoria that is highly addictive. Endorphins are 20 to 100 times more potent than morphine. Not surprising, then, that many people find exercise addictive as well.

FIGHTS COLDS AND INFECTIONS

Some exercise nuts claim they get fewer colds and bouts of flu since they began exercising, and they may be right.

Vigorous exercise produces the same therapeutic effects as a fever, according to research by two University of Michigan physiologists. Body temperature rises, which increases the efficiency of white blood cells while slowing reproduction of bacteria and viruses. The actual number of infection-fighting white blood cells in circulation increases as well. Thus exercise stimulates a bodily climate that seems to be hostile to the growth of infectious microorganisms, making us better able to fight off infections.

BUILDS BETTER BRAINS

Exercise may not only enhance heart and body-muscle activity but brain function as well. The elderly who are cardiovascularly fit experience the least memory loss.

Brisk walking exercise—even among people over age 60 who did not start out in good shape—improved reaction time and short-term memory in a study at the University of Utah.

STRENGTHENS BONES, LOOSENS STIFF JOINTS

Walking briskly can strengthen bones and minimize the brittleness and stiffness that men and women experience in later years. After age 35, women begin losing 1 to 2 percent of their bone mass every year—a process that accelerates after menopause. For men, it begins largely after age 50 or 60. But the results are the same for all of the more than 10 million people currently affected: the bones lose calcium, become demineralized, and break very easily.

Exercising seems to slow this process. If muscles around the bone are active, it stimulates the bone to acquire calcium. In one study of women with an average age of 81, those who did "chair exercises" for 30 minutes a day, 3 times a week, not only stopped the loss but actually gained calcium in their bones.

As for the joints, the stiffness that many come to expect in old age is not inevitable; much of it stems from nothing more than lack of use. If you stop rotating a joint often, through its full range of motion, the muscles, tendons, and ligaments surrounding the joint tend to tighten.

And it is often the tightening of these tissues—not any defect of the joint—that limits movement and leaves you feeling stiff.

KINDLES SEXUAL SPARKS

Increased physical activity brings about an increased interest in sex and ability to respond sexually, according to studies at the University of California and Ohio University. But it's hard to say exactly why. It may be that feeling fit simply makes one feel healthier and happier about oneself generally. Or invigorating exercise may provide just enough added energy to stoke the fires. Or improved circulation may help heighten all sensory perceptions. Whatever the reason, it seems to work. In matters like these, it may be best not to probe the whys too deeply but simply enjoy the results.

AIDS THE URGE TO QUIT SMOKING

Huffing and puffing on the track can keep you from puffing on the cigarette pack. One study showed that well over 75 percent of people who smoked when they began jogging and later went on to enter a race (in this case the 6.2 mile Peachtree Road Race in Atlanta) were able to quit smoking, and they lost weight, too.

REDUCES DIABETES

Exercise seems to improve cells' receptivity to insulin, thus reducing or even eliminating some forms of diabetes. The National Commission on Diabetes recommends exercise for many diabetes patients.

SHEDS POUNDS AND SHAPES

In addition to burning calories while you exercise, a workout speeds up your metabolism so that you continue burning extra calories for as long as fifteen to twenty-four hours afterward. Muscles also use more calories to sustain themselves than fat, so once you activate your muscles, you can eat more without gaining an ounce more than a flabby friend of the same height and weight.

Unlike dieting, which just reduces the fat all over, exercising can firm you up in specific spots, depending upon the exercises you do. Combined with dieting, it can also make the results more impressive, faster, than either endeavor can achieve alone. Muscle tissue weighs more than fat but it takes up less volume, so a fit person looks trimmer than an inactive person of the same weight.

WARDS OFF VARICOSE VEINS

Exercise that promotes steady blood circulation can help prevent the pooling of blood in limbs leading to varicose veins.

SOOTHES ANXIETY

A fifteen-minute walk is as effective a calming agent as 400 milligrams of Miltown R, a widely prescribed antianxiety agent, according to Herbert deVries, director of the physiology of exercise lab at UCLA's Andrus Gerontology Center.

For the maximum tranquilizing effect, a rhythmic exercise is best. Walking, jogging, cycling, or jumping rope all qualify.

PREVENTS THAT ACHING BACK

Back pain is *not* the price we pay for walking on two legs. About 80 percent of the 75 million Americans who suffer from back pain at some time or another have problems that do not show up on X rays. The root of the discomfort is simple and preventable: weak and overly tensed muscles that cannot provide adequate support for the spine.

Chronic bad posture seems to be the major culprit in weakening and misusing muscles. It has been found to lead not only to lower back pain but even to slipped and ruptured discs and pinched nerves.

Simple exercises can help prevent most of these common back problems. And as anyone who has ever been laid out flat for a few days knows, prevention here is critical because once your back goes out there is little anyone can do for you.

The first exercise to try, which you can do anywhere at any time, consists simply of doing what your mother nagged at you to do all through childhood—stand up straight. Or sit up straight at your desk. The trouble is that many of us don't really know what proper posture feels like.

Oddly enough, the best exercises for your back focus on your front—your abdominal muscles. Potbellies put enormous strain and pressure on the back, not simply because you're carrying extra weight but because you're throwing your spine out of proper alignment. Furthermore, the abdomen, if strong, helps keep us lifted upright and takes a lot of that muscular strain off the back muscles.

For some back exercises that will keep you supple and ease pain and strain, turn to the end of this chapter.

II. Which Exercise Is Best?

AND WHAT'S SO GREAT ABOUT AEROBICS?

All right, you've read the evidence in favor of exercising. But up until now your idea of exercise was bending down to see what's on the bottom shelf of the refrigerator, right? So what can you do to get into shape that won't kill you first?

There is only one universal measure of a good exercise—*do you do it?* If you don't enjoy the exercise enough to stick with it, no matter how good it seems, it's lousy and worthless.

To hit upon the kind of activity you'll keep up, think back to your youth and pick a sport that you used to like and feel competent doing. Be prepared for it to feel very different from what you remember; unfortunately, most sports are not like riding a bicycle and you can lose the skill. But the warm waves of nostalgia in reviving a youthful sport might just carry you through the initial stages of awkwardness to the point where you feel competent enough again to enjoy the pleasure of the movement itself. Then that pleasure, along with the recognition of how healthy you're making yourself, should keep you going after the novelty wears off.

THREE ELEMENTS OF FITNESS

In the best of all possible worlds, the activity you choose should involve the three elements critical to fitness: stretching to increase flexibility, strengthening as many muscles at the same time as possible, and increasing cardiovascular endurance through aerobic movement, which steps up the efficiency with which you can take in and distribute oxygen and relieves considerable strain on the heart.

Few activities do it all. Despite all the hoopla surrounding jogging, it is not the best all-around fitness exercise. While excellent aerobically, it does almost nothing to increase your upper body strength or your overall flexibility. However, if you add thorough warm-up and cool-down routines to your jogging, you can round out those areas that jogging misses.

Dancing and swimming can provide some of the best overall workouts. But if you repeatedly start and stop a dance class to learn new steps, you are not getting aerobic benefits. And if you swim using only one stroke, you may be benefiting only a limited group of muscles.

For the best workout, you usually have to combine several kinds of activities. Everyone, regardless of the choice of exercise, should incorporate a warm-up and cool-down series of movements into the regular routine. And you can devise your warm-up and cool-down agenda to cover precisely those areas that your main exercise misses.

THE AIM OF AEROBICS

"Aerobics" has become a household word because it is the form of exercise with the most clearly documented health benefits. If the term makes you think first of "air," you're on the right track to understanding the concept.

What you are aiming to achieve ultimately with aerobic exercise is "the training effect." It is a state in which your lungs can take in more oxygen than before—an ability that is a strong predictor of long life—and your heart can pump more efficiently, meaning it needs to beat less often to distribute the same supply of blood and oxygen throughout the body. Thus you reduce the strain on your heart when working and when resting, an effect you can measure as your resting pulse rate goes down.

For an exercise to qualify as aerobic, it should eventually increase the pulse rate for a sustained period—at least twenty minutes. Walking, swimming, biking, cross-country skiing, dancing (ballroom, folk, jazz, or exercises set to music), hiking, cycling, skating, playing squash or singles tennis can all fill the bill. Doubles tennis, bowling, and golf do not sustain the pulse rate continuously and thus don't qualify as aerobic activities, though they are certainly better than doing nothing, especially if they spur you on to other sports.

Common sense will tell you when you're giving yourself a good workout. But if you like a more systematic approach, here are the basics for understanding aerobics and achieving the training effect.

AEROBICS MADE EASY

- The maximum heart rate a healthy person should attain is 220 minus your age. So if you're 30 to 40, your maximum should be between 180 and 190.
- Your exercise heart rate—once you are in good shape—should be about 70 to 85 percent of the maximum. See the table following for a breakdown.

    If you operate at lower than the target exercise rate, you're not giving your heart as good a workout as you could; much higher, and you're exposing yourself to stress without gaining any additional fitness benefits.

    However, if you are just starting to exercise, aim for 60 percent of your maximum rate (perhaps even less—be sensible) and increase gradually.

- For optimum cardiovascular fitness, you want to sustain your target exercise rate for 20 to 30 minutes, preferably about 3 times a week, with no more than 2 days of rest in between. (Again, don't push too hard when first starting. If you're pooped after 10 minutes, cool your heels and the rest of you as well.)
- Add to that a 5-to-10-minute warm-up and 5-to-10-minute cool-down, and you'll see that a decent, safe cardiovascular workout can be done in as little as 30 minutes—90 minutes per week.

YOUR TARGET PULSE RATE

Age	Maximum Rate	Target Rate 70% to 85%	
20	200	140	170
30	190	133	162
40	180	126	153
50	170	119	145
60	160	112	136
70	150	105	128

HOW TO TAKE YOUR PULSE

You have to find two things—your pulse and a clock.

The easiest spots to find your pulse are at the wrist on the thumb side or on the side of the neck just below the jawbone.

Use your fingers, not your thumb, as the thumb has a pulse of its own.

Begin counting as soon as you stop exercising because the rate changes quickly. And count only for ten seconds, multiplying by six to get the rate for a minute, again because if you count longer, your rate will begin to fall off.

During the warm-up, you should be at about 50 percent of maximum, then you should stay at the target range of 70 to 85 percent of maximum for the middle stretch, and return to a normal pulse rate during the cool-down. The idea is basically that the fitter you are, the more you can work without dangerously elevating your pulse, and the faster your pulse will return to normal once you stop.

If you find interrupting a dance class or exercise routine to feel your throbbing veins a distracting nuisance, stop doing it. You really only need to do it a few times to check your sense of how taxing exercise is for you. It doesn't take long to develop an intuitive sense of when you're working up to speed, and then you can stop fingering your arteries and enjoy the flow of the exercise.

WHAT SHAPE ARE YOU IN?

If you're curious about how fit your cardiovascular system is, try the following tests. Just bear in mind that whatever shape you're in, you want to start any new exercise regimen slowly, to avoid possible injury and also to establish the new habits firmly.

If you are seriously overweight and out of condition, do not take the tests, just peruse the Fitness Guideline. If at any time during these tests you feel short of breath or dizzy, stop immediately.

If just thinking about exercise makes you short of breath and dizzy, carefully lift your hand and turn to chapter 11 "I-Hate-to-Exercise Exercises."

FITNESS GUIDELINE

Good condition	You can climb 3 flights of stairs and walk a fast 2 miles without having to stop and catch your breath
Fair condition	You can climb 2 flights of stairs or walk a couple of miles without huffing and puffing
Sedentary	You get out of breath after 2 flights of stairs and your pulse rate rises just thinking about having to walk 2 miles
Worse than sedentary	Going up a flight of stairs quickly leaves you breathless and a half-mile walk sends your heart thumping hard

THE HOP TEST

Take your pulse at rest. For most people it is between 60 and 80.

Then hop 25 times on one foot and 25 times on the other. Take your pulse immediately. If it goes up more than 50 points, you are not in terribly good shape.

Sit for 2 minutes. Take your pulse again. It should be within 5 to 10 points of your resting pulse. The further off you are, the less fit you are.

FITNESS GUIDELINE

OK shape	Resting pulse—between 60 and 80 First pulse was less than 50 points above resting pulse Second pulse should come within 5 to 10 points of resting pulse
Poor shape	Resting pulse much higher than 80—it means your heart is working hard First pulse went higher than 50 above your resting pulse Second pulse remained more than 10 points higher than resting pulse

FLEXIBILITY TEST

Sit on the floor with your legs stretched out straight in front of you a couple of inches apart. Place a ruler on the floor between your legs so the 6-inch mark is at your heels and the 12-inch mark is farthest away from your body.

Keep your back straight, feet flexed, and gently and slowly bend over, reaching as far as you can on the ruler. Do not bounce forward, and do not slump your back and shoulders.

Men are often stiffer and less flexible here than women. All of us can improve this flexibility by gentle stretching movements. Try this before you have warmed up or worked out, then again afterward. You should see considerable difference.

Your Touch Point	Flexibility Rating
Can't touch it	Stiff, need to stretch
1–3	Not so bad, but limbering wouldn't hurt
4–6	Good
7–10	Very Good
11 or more	Excellent, but don't stop exercising or you can become stiff again

EXERCISES THROUGH THE AGES—YOUTH, MIDDLE, AND OLDER YEARS

There is some form of exercise that will make us healthy and fit at every age. And there is also some form that will be dangerous, for the very young supple bodies as well as the older, brittler bones.

One thing that does not change with age or stages of fitness or kind of exercise is that you should do a warm-up routine before setting out and a cool-down routine at the end, each lasting at least five or ten minutes. These will not only decrease your chances of injury but maximize your chances for a well-rounded workout.

KIDS' EXERCISE—DOS AND DON'TS

We are learning that children can do more mentally and physically at younger ages than we ever thought possible. By age one week, a baby can pick her mother's voice from among a medley of voices. By four to five months a child can remember faces for two weeks that he was exposed to for only ninety seconds. With physical skills, too, it has become clear that children can develop their gripping strength and crawling and walking abilities much earlier if allowed to explore instead of being confined in strollers, infant seats, and playpens. YMCAs across the country have introduced exercise and swimming classes for six-month-olds. The new childhood education message is that children, from the first week of life, can and should be stimulated to feel the pleasure of movement.

But there is a risk that we can go overboard. If we introduce activities that are too advanced for the child's motor coordination, we will simply frustrate the child. Or worse, we may even doom her to failure and make her give up on all sports.

Balance is as crucial in one's approach to children's exercise as it is in the physical execution of the exercise. So here are a few cautionary notes on specific kinds of exercise for children.

Team sports. While being on a team can teach subtle lessons about competition and cooperation, it can also teach not-so-subtle lessons about the frailty of children's bodies. Protective equipment is critical. Good shoes for support, protective gear for head, face, and eyes must be worn.

Too rigorous exercise—from running track, soccer, or dancing— can damage children's growth plates, which are groups of specialized cells at either end of long bones that cause bone growth. So even though children seem more flexible, they, too, need to warm up slowly and should not be allowed to play with any injury.

Long-distance running. Don't do it advises the American Academy of Pediatrics. Children under sixteen should never attempt a full adult marathon. They can get heel-cord injuries and chronic joint trauma. They do not adapt to temperature extremes while running long distances as well as adults. And further, they can suffer psychological problems if they set unrealistic goals for themselves or if they feel pressured by parents.

Ballet. Students shouldn't use pointe shoes until age ten to twelve, or they risk traumatic arthritis and damage to growth plates.

Swimming. It's a fine sport for all ages, even children under age three, as long as the emphasis with toddlers is on enjoying the water, not on learning to swim.

MIDDLERS

Start slowly. No piece of advice is more important, and less heeded. Older folks know this caution all too well, and the youngsters have resilient enough bones and muscles that even if they forget, their bodies usually forgive. But those in the middle tend to let initial enthusiasm outrun common sense, and in addition to pain you are asking for ultimate defeat. Once you're in pain or injured, you're more likely to quit for good. And then where will you be?

There need not be pain. If you increase your pace gradually—

whether running, walking, dancing—you can not only avoid injury but eliminate that painful stage. Sure, muscles may ache a little the day after. But if there is pain while you're working out, it usually means you're pushing too hard.

And if you wake up the day after with sore muscles, don't give in and skip your workout. If you at least make yourself do some gentle stretching exercises, you'll feel more limber and less achy afterward.

ELDERLY

Who needs physician approval before beginning?

Perhaps 1 percent of men below thirty-five and 10 percent above that age may have hidden heart disease, according to the American Heart Association. Even for most of these people, exercise will not be harmful. But just to be safe, all elderly, or anyone with known risks for heart disease—family history, diabetes, heavy smoking, high blood pressure—should discuss with a physician whether they need an exercise stress test before beginning a new regimen. Even those who have had heart attacks can still engage in rigorous physical activity if they have built up to it slowly under supervision. A group of Canadians, all of whom had suffered heart attacks, got together several years back, dubbed themselves "the sickest track club in the world," and successfully completed the Boston Marathon (26 miles, 385 yards) under the guidance of their doctor, Dr. Terence Kavanaugh.

The older you get, the less rigorous activity you need to reach your target pulse rate and thus get your cardiovascular system in shape. So walk before you run.

WALKING VERSUS RUNNING

Running addicts will tell you that all sorts of wonderful things have happened since they began running—they've lost weight, given up smoking, feel fitter and more cheerful and happier.

It's all true, but what they don't tell you is how many times they've hurt themselves. A study of Peachtree Road Race runners by the Centers for Disease Control showed that more than a third of the runners in that ten-kilometer race developed some knee or foot problem within a year of the race. Four percent also reported dog bites, and a few had been hit by bikes or cars.

The latest evidence suggests that while running may reap all sorts of health benefits, brisk walking will, too—without most of the problems and injuries.

The foot is a complex piece of machinery composed of 26 bones, 33 muscles, and 56 ligaments. Pressure on any of these points transfers directly from the foot to the legs, hips, and back. The energy transfer is highly efficient—none of the pounding pressure is lost. When you run, the foot strikes 1500 times in an hour, exerting a shock that is four to five times greater than when you walk. All these factors provide considerable opportunity for missteps and strain during a run.

Carrying an attaché case or a heavy purse while you walk can make you fitter even faster. A group that walked about 3 miles per hour for 30 minutes a day carrying 6.6-pound backpacks (that's a good but not terribly brisk walking pace carrying a weight lighter than most attaché cases) for 3 weeks improved their cardiovascular fitness considerably—over 15 percent in three weeks. The improvement was 30 percent if in the fourth week they doubled the weight of their load during the walk. Improvement was greatest among those who started off in the worst shape.

Another study had people walking 2 to 3 miles per hour for 40 minutes a day 4 times a week without backpacks. And they improved their aerobic fitness by 28 percent in 20 weeks.

In short, walking can do the trick—the faster you walk and the more you carry, obviously the speedier the fitness results. And walking burns up almost as many calories as running—jogging a mile in 8.5 minutes burns up only about 25 more calories than walking a mile in 12 minutes.

Furthermore, the gentle rhythm of walking, in addition to soothing an anxious soul, also allows you to sustain a continuous line of thought—even a conversation—while working out.

Instead of being dismissed as "too easy," this time-honored activity should be taken seriously for that very reason. Being easy, it is an activity that you are least likely to abandon. Anyone can do it, at any age, nearly anywhere, any time, *for free*.

III. How to Keep It Up Once You've Begun

More than half of those who start an exercise program, even those who know they should keep it up because they have serious coronary risks, drop out after three to six months.

Why? How can you be one of those who, at last, sticks to it?

Here are some tips gathered from the latest behavioral research on what can successfully motivate the wary and the downright obstinate to exercise.

KEEP IT UP

The advice that follows can be applied to any kind of behavior change you want to make and stick to, not just exercising but dieting, quitting smoking, starting a daily relaxation session, or changing any other routine habits.

1. Set very simple, specific, and easily obtainable goals at first.

   Don't say, "I'm going to run around the block tomorrow." Start out by saying, "Tomorrow, I'm going to put on my running shoes. Then next week, I'll put on my running shoes and check out the block, maybe run, maybe walk, but at least go around it."

   It may sound silly. But exercisers who don't meet their goals drop out twice as fast as those who do, no matter how simple or difficult the goals. You're not doing yourself any good by setting impressive goals that you can't meet and soon abandon. If you go easy on yourself, starting modestly, you're more likely to finish with impressive improvements.

2. Pick out a special "exercise outfit" that you use for nothing else.

   It doesn't have to be jazzy or designed exclusively for the sport you choose, though it may help if you feel as though you look good in it. The point is that the outfit helps put you in the mood for exercise. It's like a signal that a hypnotist uses or you can use to put yourself in a relaxed state (see chapter 12, "Learning to Love Stress," for more on self-hypnosis and the stress fix)—whenever you see it or put it on, you immediately think of your exercise routine and you feel like moving.

3. Try a group activity.

   The vast majority of people benefit from the social support of a group. If there is a set time and place already scheduled for your exercise, it is harder to skip it than if you're on your own. The group can also spur you on to try just a little bit harder. Besides, the huffing and puffing of others helps drown out your own heavy breathing.

   If selecting a group exercise, pick a small class in which you can get some individual attention. One study of people who walked or jogged for two days a week for twelve weeks showed that those who had gotten individual praise, not simply the standard group praise at the end of a session, were more likely to be sticking to the regimen three months later.

4. Pick a location of a class or a track close to home or work; and pay in advance.

If the place is too far away and you have to make too many changes in your behavior to get there, chances are greater that you won't make it. Advance payment provides further incentive to attend all sessions of a dance, exercise, or tennis class.

5. Enlist the support of your spouse or friend.

Studies show that backup from your spouse and loved ones makes you twice as likely to keep it up.

6. Keep track of your progress.

Record in a log each time you exercise and try to pinpoint some of the improvements you have made. Improvements don't have to be simply moving faster or farther but can also be noticing how much easier a movement was or how enjoyable and refreshing the workout felt.

7. Reward yourself often.

Not just for making clear-cut improvements but for sticking to the routine each week. Pick a treat that pleases you but that also is linked somehow to the aim of the exercises. For example, if you're using exercise to help you relax, reward yourself by going to see a movie. If food is a better motivator, instead of a slice of cake, treat yourself to an excellent, healthy meal.

8. Keep off the scales.

Even though you're burning calories, you're not likely to see quick weight loss, and getting on the scales to check will only be disappointing. If you need something to measure, get a calipers and measure the change in body fat—that is also a more important measurement than weight. But here, too, don't expect big results for four to eight weeks.

9. Take your pulse.

Within the first month, you may see a drop of as much as ten points in your resting pulse. This means you are getting fitter, your heart is getting stronger, you're reducing stress, and all this exercising is worth keeping up.

10. Know that you will relapse at some point and prepare for it.

With any attempt at changing behavior—from dieting to quitting smoking to starting exercising—the question is not whether you'll give up at some point, but when.

Have a plan for when the impulse to pack it in hits. Try to set a limit on the number of days or weeks you will allow to slip by before getting back in the exercise swing. Remember that exercising isn't an all-or-nothing proposition. You have not failed because you missed a session, or two, or more. You started up once and you can and will start up again. So if a vacation, or a business trip, or an injury, or just sagging spirits gets you out of the rhythm, just tell yourself it was inevitable. It had to happen sooner or later. And then get going again.

EXERCISE AND BURNING CALORIES

Most people are surprised at how few calories exercise actually burns up. For example, it takes about fifteen minutes of continuous jogging to burn up the calories in one martini. Still, if one engagesn as much activity as possible throughout the day, every day, the gains can be considerable losses in unwanted fat by the end of a few months.

Activity	Calories Burned Per Half Hour
Mopping floors or vacuuming Walking leisurely (3 mph) Cycling at a calm pace	135
Ballet or dance exercises Doubles tennis Scrubbing floors	165
Walking briskly (4 mph) Cycling briskly Roller or ice skating Water skiing	200
Singles tennis Swimming Downhill skiing	225
Squash, handball Jogging (over 5 mph) Cycling vigorously	320

BACK EXERCISES

Back pain takes most people by surprise. You go along thinking everything is fine, not particularly conscious of your body one way or the other, believing it will continue to serve you happily without any special treatment. Then you do something "funny," something that you've done a hundred times, something that doesn't seem terribly demanding—you sneeze, you lift your child in the middle of the night, you bend over to make the bed, pull a weed, or pick up a book—and *blam*. There's a twinge, a searing pain. The slightest movement sends a terrifying electrical current of torture through your back to your hips, legs, arms. You lie flat on your back, trying desperately not to move by accident and tempt that shock again, but sooner or later your nose itches, or you have to cough, or you simply take a deep breath, and the pain crashes over you like an ink-black wave, erasing every thought but *pain.*

It can happen to anyone at any time; it does not take any unusual activity to trigger it. Back pain usually results from an accumulation of strains over a long period—your back takes the first 1000 strains but number 1001 proves just too much. It is that straw that broke the camel's back. But it is not that straw at all that is to blame, or even the thousands of straws piled up before. For most of us camels, what "breaks" our backs is not so much overuse as underuse and misuse, not doing what we can to protect our backs in advance.

Cultivating strength and flexibility is the best safeguard against back troubles. Both back and stomach muscles must be strong enough to support your weight as you move, but they must also be supple enough to give with the unpredictable bursts of activity that life occasionally demands.

ARE YOU HEADED FOR TROUBLE?

How can you tell if you're strong and supple enough?

Lie flat on your back. Now, if you cannot do a sit-up, or raise both legs a foot off the floor and hold that position for 10 seconds, then your stomach muscles are too weak to support your body weight and you're asking for back trouble.

If you cannot lie flat on your front, lift your legs and hold them straight out for 10 seconds, your back muscles are dangerously weak.

And if you cannot bend over with straight legs and touch the floor with your fingertips, the problem is not that your legs are too long or your arms too short, but rather tension has tightened and shortened your back and hamstring muscles, reducing their critical suppleness and flexibility.

No matter how old you are, or how long it's been since you've exercised, you can improve muscle strength and flexibility. These exercises focus not only on the back but the abdomen and other muscles essential to the support of the back. Even if you are already in good overall shape, these exercises are important because other activities— like running, or tennis, or dancing—do not always isolate and tone these critical muscle groups.

Begin slowly with a gentle warm-up. If you already have a history of back trouble, you want to proceed especially slowly with consultation from a physician or back specialist.

NECK LIMBERER

Head rolls. This limbers up the neck and the shoulder muscles that help support the top of the spine.

Stand with your feet hip-width (about a foot) apart, stomach in, spine long, shoulders relaxed and down, hands hanging loosely at your sides.

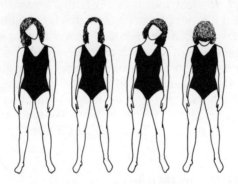

Slowly drop your chin to your chest, roll your head to the right shoulder (moving nothing but the head) letting the full 15 pounds of head weight stretch your neck as you continue the smooth roll back and to the left and front again.

Roll 4 times to the right, then 4 times to the left. Concentrate on a full rotation; resist the tendency to let your shoulders hunch up—keep them down and open wide; and although you are relaxed, keep stomach muscles firm at all times.

BACK LIMBERER

Cat stretches. These cat stretches are excellent for relieving tension, limbering the back, and easing mild lower back pain.

Kneel on all fours, with your knees planted directly below your hip joints, hip-width apart, and your hands planted in line with your shoulders, so you form a sturdy rectangle.

Concentrate on your stomach and buttock muscles and let them lead the movement.

Tighten the stomach and tuck the pelvis and buttocks under as you simultaneously let the head drop down and arch your back to make an upside down U out of your body.

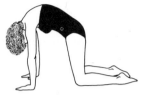

Reverse the U by releasing the buttocks, pointing them toward the ceiling as you also lift the head and let the back sink. Feel the release, the stretch.

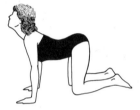

Then repeat.

Move slowly, smoothly, gently stretching each part of you like a cat.

STOMACH

Modified bicycle. Lie on your back with knees bent and feet flat on the floor, arms straight by your sides.

Inhale, then exhale as you slowly and steadily lift your head and lift your right knee, trying to bring your forehead to your knee. The movement should be smooth, not jerky.

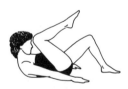

Inhale as you gently return foot and head to the floor; repeat with the other knee, and alternate 10 times. Rest and do it again, if you can. Increase the number as you get stronger.

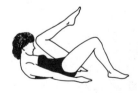

Bicycle. This is slightly more rigorous than the above.

Stretch out flat on the floor, fold your hands behind your head. As you lift your head up, bend your knees and touch your right elbow to your left knee.

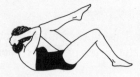

Then stretch out flat again on floor.

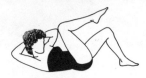

Repeat movement touching left elbow to right knee.

Later, when you have gotten used to this exercise, you can increase the difficulty by raising the outstretched leg off the floor while the other leg bends to meet the elbow, and alternating elbow-knee touches without lying back in between.

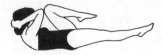

Don't forget to breathe throughout. Take small breaths and exhale in short puffs as you reach to touch elbow to knee.

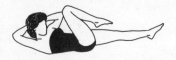

STOMACH AND BACK STRENGTHENER

Slow-Motion Sit-ups. These sit-ups are not the usual variety, so pay attention. There is no such thing as "men's sit-ups" and "women's sit-ups"—there's a right way and a wrong way. And the old way, often called "men's," with straight legs and a jerking motion to lift you up, can strain your back.

If done slowly and properly (which is harder than doing them fast), these sit-ups will strengthen stomach muscles and limber the spine.

Lie down with knees up, arms by your sides.

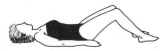

Concentrate on your deep abdominal muscles before moving.

Use those muscles to roll up gently to a sitting position, rolling through one vertebra at a time up the spine. Use your arms for leverage if you need to.

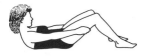

Sit up straight, stomach still in.

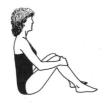

Then roll down in a slow, controlled movement, curling so the small of the back makes contact with the floor first, followed by each vertebra up the spine as you straighten and lengthen and relax.

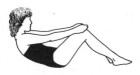

Repeat until you can no longer do the movement smoothly. If you find at any point as you lift up that you are jerking yourself up, rather than lifting up in a continuous, fluid movement, then you are using your back, not your stomach muscles, and that defeats the point of the exercise. Rest and try again.

Warm-Up/Cool-Down Routines

No one likes to be thrown into new circumstances cold, least of all your muscles. No matter how fit you are, warming up slowly before you begin a workout will reduce your chances of pulling, tearing, or straining tendons, ligaments, and muscles.

Cooling down for several minutes after a workout is important, too. If you come to an abrupt halt after running or playing ball or dancing, you may get dizzy and even faint, because your leg muscles are no longer helping to pump your blood but allowing it to pool in your legs. Runners should walk, dancers should walk, everyone who has had an aerobic workout should walk to unwind. When your breathing and pulse have returned to normal, then it is an ideal time to take advantage of your warmed-up body to do a few extra stretching and toning movements for muscles your exercise may have overlooked. And finally, the cool-down should slow the pace further, relax the entire body, and bring the workout to a graceful, peaceful close.

WARM-UP

Breath lift. Inhale deeply as you lift your arms straight out to your sides, stretching through the fingertips, and up to the ceiling.

Exhale as you bring your arms back down to your sides.

Repeat five times.

Head rolls. Stand with your feet hip distance (about a foot) apart. Let your head fall gently forward, chin on chest, and roll your head to the right, back, around to the left and front again. Continue to the right for 4 rotations.

Repeat to the left for 4 rotations.

Shoulder lifts. Stand up straight. Lift both shoulders to the ears and ease them back down, twice. Then lift the right shoulder and release, lift the left shoulder and release.

Repeat that entire sequence 5 times. (Throw in a shoulder roll if you want to try something a little jazzier than a simple shoulder lift.)

Side stretch. Stand with legs about 2 feet apart. Reach your right arm over your head with fingers reaching toward the left and stretch; stay in that position (stomach in, spine long) and pulse gently—do not bounce—3 times. Stand up straight on the fourth beat.

Repeat the stretch with the left arm overhead leaning right. Pulse 3 times. Come up.

Repeat the sequence 4 times.

Waist twists. Stand with legs wide (more than 2 feet) apart, arms out to the side at shoulder height.

With legs straight, turn your upper body to the right as far as you can go, then to the left. Try to look to the back wall or farther each time. Do this in a slow, controlled movement or you can hurt your back.

Repeat 10 times.

Bends. Stand with feet wide apart. Bend over, keeping your legs straight, and let your hands touch the floor (between your feet or behind you if you can reach farther) and the weight of your head pull you down. Let the head dangle loosely.

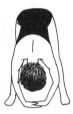

Now move your body over your right foot and hang down, reaching your hands as far beyond that foot as possible. Hold.

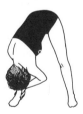

Reach over to the left side and hold.

Back to center, keep your head dangling down, and return slowly to a standing position, rolling up one vertebra at a time.

Repeat the sequence. As you get limberer, you can try grabbing hold of the ankle and gently pulling your chest to your thigh.

Calf stretch. Stand with feet together. Stretch your right foot directly behind a distance of about 2 feet, keeping both heels on the floor at all times. Bend the front leg and stretch the back calf, keeping back straight, stomach in, and, again, both feet flat on floor. Bend your front knee and straighten 5 times in a gentle fluid movement.

Bring feet together.

Repeat on the left side.

Alternate stretches 4 times.

Finger press. Warming up the hands is important for any racquet or ball sport that uses them. Dancers, too, need to awaken their finger muscles. Many exercise routines overlook the hands, so this is also good to do after a workout, in the cool-down routine.

Hold hands up about a foot in front of your chest, spread your fingers wide and bring the fingertips together, pressing strongly. Your elbows should be pointing out to the side walls and pulling outward against the pressure of the fingers. (Don't let those shoulders creep up toward your ears.)

This isometric exercise involves concentrating on pulling outward with the elbows and pressing together with the fingers simultaneously. It is good for your hands, chest, shoulders, and upper back.

Hamstring stretch. Sit down, legs stretched out in a V to the sides. Keep your back straight as you lean forward between your legs to the floor, stretching the back of the legs—do not bounce. Let the weight of your head and arms ease you down. Hold 8 counts.

Come up, face right, and gently lean over your right leg, keeping both buttocks on the floor and both legs straight. Hold, exhale, and try to relax and stretch farther, for 8 counts.

Repeat to the left.

Then repeat the entire sequence.

Slow-motion run. You are not trying to run yet; this is more of a springy jump. Simply stand with your weight on your left foot and jump to your right foot, landing on your toes and working slowly through the toes, ball, and heel of your foot as the foot flattens on the floor. Jump to the left foot and repeat, alternating feet.

After the feet are warmed up, build to a run in place.

COOL-DOWN

Run in place. Run in place, slowing to a walk, as long as it takes for your breath and pulse to return to normal.

Bends. Bend over with straight back, reach your hands through your legs toward the back wall and swing through your legs 5 times.

Now turn to the right, bending over the right leg and proceed to stretch as in the Bends exercise of the Warm-up.

Sit-ups. Very few exercise regimens give the stomach muscles enough of a workout. A few sit-ups can't hurt, if you do them right.

Do bent-knee Slow-Motion Sit-ups.

Advanced bicycles. Again, if you want to avert back troubles and cultivate beautiful posture, work on those abdominal muscles.

Lie on your back with legs out straight, hands behind the head. Lift right knee and left elbow to meet above belly button as left leg stays straight a few inches off the floor; then bring right elbow to left knee. Repeat 20 times.

For detailed description of this movement and variations see the Modified Bicycle and Bicycle stomach exercises.

Buttocks tucks. For a description of this movement, turn to the While Doing Dishes exercises in Chapter 11.

Cat stretches. Again, this will limber up the back. See the Back Limberer described earlier.

Plow. This is a yoga stretch for the back, shoulders, and neck.

Lie on your back, roll up to a shoulder stand, then drop your feet over your head to the floor behind you (or as far as they'll go), letting your knees rest around your ears if they reach that far. Hold.

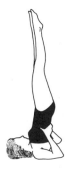
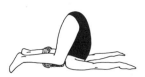

Now straighten your legs and reach your toes to the wall behind you. Then release and let your knees rest near your ears again. Straighten legs, and release. Hold.

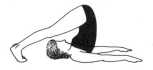

Then roll back down, slowly, feeling each vertebra make contact with the floor.

Face stretch. Now, lying flat on your back, stretch your face muscles—most of us forget about that part of our body.

Stick your tongue out, smile as hard as you can, scream silently, or aloud if you want, tensing your cheeks, opening your jaw, squinting your eyes. Now release it all. Blow your cheeks wide as if they were a bubble—that loosens the jaw. Now release. (Repeat if you want to; it feels great.)

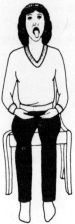

Now feel your entire body sink, relaxed, into the floor. Close your eyes. Take two deep breaths. Exhale slowly.

Good work.

11
I-Hate-to-Exercise Exercises

*A Plan for Those Who Dislike the Whole Idea
or Just Can't Seem to Find the Time*

DON'T GET UP. You can take this test without a pencil.

If you agree with any of the following statements, then you don't even need to lift your page-flipping fingers—this chapter's for you.

1. Everybody told me exercise would feel great, but all I felt was damp and smelly.
2. I have allergies—you can't run and sneeze at the same time. Besides how can you possibly get healthy running outside in this air?
3. I never was good at sports as a kid and I never enjoyed them, so why should I go out of my way to humiliate myself at my age?
4. I have a terrific-looking exercise outfit; it seems silly to mess it up by actually *working out* in it.
5. There aren't enough hours in the day as it is, I'm already pooped by evening, and you want me to try to jam in exercising, too? What are you, crazy?

Don't throw the eclair. There will be no mention of the dread word "exercise," not exactly anyway. The problem is that you've been thinking of exer . . . , you know, as some isolated activity that you have to dress up (or down) for and go to some special facility to do.

The truth is that life is exercise (that was the last mention). And exercise (no, honestly, this is really the last time) is simply movement.

You have to move at some point every day, even if it is only from the bed to the car. So you may as well make the most of the moves you have to make. You can use them to get you in shape without spending extra time, money, or effort.

If you're feeling low on energy, you're overweight, you smoke a lot and cough, too, you'd rather sit than move. The only problem is that the more you sit, the stiffer your bones and joints get and the less you feel like moving. Then when you do move, you feel old and crotchety. You act old and crotchety. You get treated as if you're old and crotchety. And pretty soon, no matter how young your birth certificate says you are, *you will be old and crotchety.*

Sure, you're sick and tired of hearing all this gushy talk about physical fitness and watching an endless stream of musclemen and pencil-thin women parade across the television screen urging you to work out. It's enough to make a person roll over and go back to sleep. But if you also wish there were a way to feel better without having to jog or roll around on a gym floor, the tips here will come in handy.

All the movements that follow are things you can do anywhere at any time, while sitting or standing, in bed or in the shower, at your desk or at the sink, watching television or waiting in a line. They will tone and strengthen muscles while relieving aches and pains and stiffness.

You don't need special equipment or any skill. They'll help you begin to enjoy moving instead of dreading it. And pretty soon, since movement begets movement, you may find yourself actually wanting to do more. You'll feel oddly energetic, strong, limber, and cheerful.

OK, maybe "cheerful" went too far. But stranger things have happened. Take the risk. Start small. Keep your eyelid muscles working and read on.

Stretch While Reading

THE BOOK STRETCH
Good for the arms, back, and waist.
1. Sit up straight, feet flat on the floor, stomach in, back straight, shoulders down.
2. Hold the book open in both hands and straighten your arms in front of you, keeping your shoulders down and your arms at shoulder height.
3. Keep your eyes on the middle of the page, your feet and knees pointing front, and move the book slowly 90 degrees to the right, so you're stretching at the waist and the back. Hold and read 5 sentences.

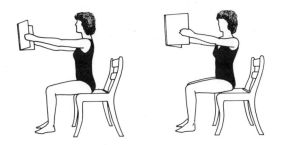

4. Now bring your arms back in front of you and repeat the stretch to the left.
5. Repeat 5 times.

In and Out of the Shower

SHOWER STRETCH
Limbers shoulders, neck, back, and arms.
1. Simply reach your arms to the ceiling, stretching the right side, then the left, in smooth rhythmic pulses as the hot soothing water further warms up your muscles.
2. Reach 10 times on each side.

SOAP UP
Limbers the legs and back.
1. With legs straight and back straight and stomach held firmly, bend over slowly, then let the back round and the head hang loosely.
2. Hang and stretch (do not bounce) as you lather up your hands with soap.

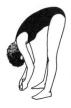 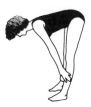

3. Now straighten the back, begin soaping up your left ankle, knee, thigh, on up as you lift slowly, keeping the back straight until you're standing.
4. Repeat so you can soap up the other side.

DRY OFF

Good for the leg and stomach muscles—you can do this not only while drying, but while applying moisture lotion or, for women, while shaving the legs.

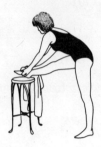

1. Make sure one leg is planted firmly on a nonslip towel or rug, toes pointing straight ahead, as you lift the other leg onto the counter or toilet seat or stool and slightly to the side. Keep both supporting leg and raised leg straight. Bend over with stomach in and back straight, and dry each toe thoroughly, then move up the leg and straighten and dry the rest of your right side, keeping the leg in place.
2. Stand up straight, hold stomach in firmly, and lift the outstretched leg a couple of inches above the counter and then back down to the floor.
3. Repeat on the other side.

At the Desk

TRIANGLE STRETCH

Limbers and strengthens shoulders, arms, and hands

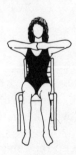

1. Clasp fingers in front of your chest (one palm faces you, the other faces so that fingers can grip and pull in opposite directions). Hold the arms parallel to the floor, with the elbows forming 2 points of a large triangle. (The third point is the vertebra at the base of the neck.)
2. Pull fingers in opposite directions. Feel the elbows pointing outward in opposite directions as well. Stretch and hold. Release. Repeat with hands clasped the other way.
3. Turn to the right, repeat the stretch.
4. Turn left and repeat.
5. Lift hands above the head and repeat the stretch.

In the Chair

CHAIR STRETCH
Limbers the back, and can be done in a bus, plane, or train as well as the office.

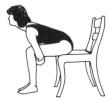

1. Sit on the edge of your chair, lean over and rest your chest on your thighs, your hands on your toes or the floor in front of you.
2. Wrap your arms underneath your knees, right hand clasping left elbow and left elbow clasping right. Now try to sit up and stretch gently. Hold. Release and go back down on your chest.
3. Then immediately straighten the back from the lower back to the top of the head, and come up to sitting slowly.
4. Repeat 5 times.

CHAIR PRESS
Strengthens the arms, chest, and back; the advanced version also strengthens stomach and leg muscles.

1. If you have a very strong armchair, rest your hands on the arms of the chair and lift yourself up completely out of the chair. Hold 2 counts. Lower yourself back to sitting. Repeat 5 times.

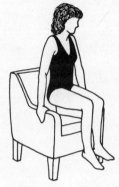

2. Advanced chair press: point your legs straight out first, then lift yourself up.

LEG LIFTS
Strengthens and tones the legs and stomach.
1. Sit close to the edge of a sturdy chair. With back straight and stomach muscles prepared to work, point your toes, lift both feet slightly off the floor, then extend both legs straight out in front of you at hip height.

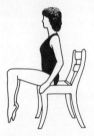
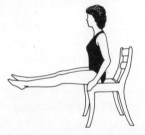

2. Hold 5 seconds.
3. Bend at the knees with toes still pointed, and gently rest the feet back on the floor.
4. Repeat 5 times. As you get stronger, try stretching and bending and then stretching again before you rest. Increase the number of stretches between rests gradually.

At the Copier

PUSH-UPS
Tones the arms, chest, stomach muscles. You can also do these against the wall.

1. Stand 3 to 4 feet from the copying machine, keep feet flat on the floor, back straight, and lean over, placing both hands on the edge.

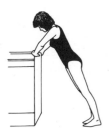 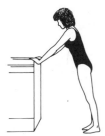

2. Push up until your arms are straight. Keep both legs straight as well.
3. Repeat 10 times.
4. Now stand on your toes and repeat 10 times.

On the Phone

PHONE STRETCH

Stretches and tones the arms and the chest muscles.

1. Hold the phone to your left ear with your right hand. Now lift your free left hand, stretching straight up in the air, rotate the hand out to the side, then reach straight-armed as far behind you as you can as if you were trying to get your arm to extend straight out your back. Push 5 times, stretching your arm behind you. Then bring the arm back out to the side, then stretch it up to the ceiling and down to grasp the phone.

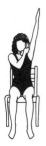 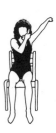

2. Switch phone to other hand and repeat on the other side.
3. Better yet, do the above exercise holding your tape dispenser or another light weight.

LEG KICKS
Good for the stomach and legs and back.
1. Sit on the edge of your chair with hands on the seat beside you. Lift up heels, kick right foot straight out in front of you, slowly enough to straighten the leg fully, keeping the right knee as high as the left. Bring the foot back. Repeat with the left leg. Repeat 20 times.

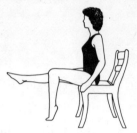

2. Remember throughout to point your toes, keep your back straight and your stomach sucked in.

LEG KICKS 2
1. Sit on the edge of your chair with hands on the seat beside you.
2. Kick your leg out, point the toe, then flex, then point and flex again.
3. Then change legs and repeat.
4. Repeat the entire sequence 20 times.

Waiting in Line

FOOT FLEXES/FOOT CIRCLES
Good for developing good posture and balance as well as limbering ankles and toning stomach, buttock, and leg muscles.

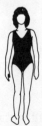

1. Stand up straight, shoulders down, stomach in, and extend right leg in front of you. Balance.

2. Now flex the foot strongly, then point, flex and point 5 times. (When this gets easy, try foot circles—circling the ankles to the right 5 times and then to the left 5 times.)
3. Extend the leg out to the right and do 5 sets of flex points (or circles).

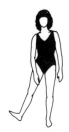 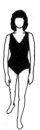

4. Extend the leg straight out behind you, keeping your back straight and pelvis and buttocks tucked slightly underneath you (don't lean forward or let the pelvis tilt back), and do the foot flexes (or circles).
5. Change legs and repeat the sequence on the other side.

SLOW-MOTION WALK

Good for stretching ankles and calves and thighs; excellent for lines that seem to be moving nowhere. This is the mime walk in which you look as if you're walking but are actually staying in the same spot. It takes more muscle control and coordination than running in place. And it is actually easier to do than to explain.

1. Stand with your left foot flat on the floor and your right foot stretched forward, flexed as if you are about to plant your heel down and take a step.

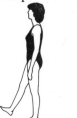 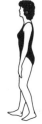

2. Instead of walking onto the right, lift up slightly onto the ball of your left foot just enough so you can slide your right foot back along the floor until the right toes are even with the left.

3. Now stretch your left foot out, flexed, as if about to take a step. Lift up onto the ball of your right foot and drag the left foot back (heel lightly dragging along the floor, foot still flexed) until it is even with the right.

4. Repeat until you get the hang of it.

RUN IN PLACE
Good for the legs as well as the cardiovascular system.
1. Keep your stomach pulled in, back straight, chin up.
2. Now run in place, lifting your knees high, landing on the balls of your feet and working through to the heel on each step.

While Washing Dishes

BUTTOCKS TUCKS
Good for strengthening buttocks, lower back, and stomach. You can do this standing or sitting—especially good to do while driving or waiting in line in winter when winter coats allow you to proceed discreetly.

1. With feet about hip distance apart, tighten the buttocks and pull the pelvis slightly forward. Release.
2. Repeat as long as you can—or until the dishes are done.

HIP SWINGS
Good for limbering hip joints, and strengthening lower back and stomach.
1. With your feet hip distance apart (about a foot), stomach in and back straight, bend your knees slightly, and swing your hips to the right and then the left, keeping the upper part of the body still.
2. Repeat smoothly—no jerking—for 16 counts.
3. Then swing pelvis forward toward the sink and backward, again keeping the legs bent but the back as straight as possible.

Make these movements fluid and rhythmical—they are sexy and they are good for you—so enjoy them.

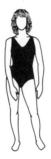

TV Toning

COMMERCIAL FACE STRETCH
Limbers the face, releases tension in the forehead and jaw, and wards off tension headaches.
1. During the commercials, instead of drooling at the food ads, open your mouth as wide as you can, stick your tongue out, squinch your eyes up, and stretch every muscle in your face. Release and repeat until your family cracks up.

LEG LIFTS
Tones the legs, stomach, and back, and you can keep on watching the tube all the while.
1. Get on your hands and knees, making a rectangle with those four points—hands directly under the shoulders, knees under the hip joints.

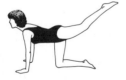 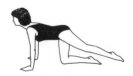

2. Stretch your left leg straight out behind you, point your toes, now lift and lower, lift and lower. Repeat 10 times. Now turn the leg out in the hip socket, flex the foot, and repeat the same thing 10 times.
3. Change legs and repeat.

DONKEY KICKS
Tones and trims the hips and thighs.
1. Get on your hands and knees (as you did for leg lifts). Lift your

right knee up behind you, flex your foot, and get your heel as high as you can. Now kick your leg out and pull your heel back to your buttocks. Repeat 20 times.

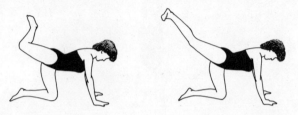

2. Repeat on the left side. Remember to keep stomach in, back straight, shoulders down, and chin up.

ELBOW-KNEE TOUCHES

Good for the stomach and the back and the legs. You can do this lying down or even sitting down.

1. Clasp your hands behind your head. Lift the right knee and touch it with the left elbow. While lowering right knee, lift the left knee and touch it with the right elbow. And so on.
2. Repeat 20 times. Keep stomach muscles tight the entire time.

The Good Posture Exercise—The Foundation on Which All Else Is Built

Simply standing up straight—if you do it right—is, in itself, an excellent toning movement for the chest, shoulder, stomach, and back muscles.

Good posture is a great boon to good health. The correct, natural stance not only makes you look good but it also allows you to move with the most poise and balance and the least muscular effort.

Fundamental though it may be, many of us don't really know what good posture looks or feels like. Even those who are active and agile are not always conscious of the best way to hold their bodies when at rest. And the example most of us think of first when posture is mentioned—the military posture, with chin up, chest out, and shoulders pressed back—is as bad for you as slouching.

Externally, you are aiming to create the longest, straightest (though not rigid) line from head to toe, seen from all angles, front, back, and side.

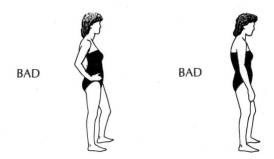

BAD   BAD

Internally, you are aiming to use only those muscles necessary to lengthen and widen the midsection so that the spine is supported (by the stomach as well as the back muscles), the internal organs are not cramped, and the lungs can inflate fully and easily.

As you follow these instructions, stand with your side to a full-length mirror so you can see what you usually do—and what you really should be doing. The right way may not feel "natural" at first, so it will take some adjusting.

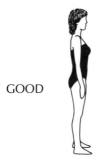

GOOD

1. Stand with your feet about an inch apart and your weight planted evenly on both feet, neither on your heels nor on your toes. Rock ever so gently forward onto the ball of your foot, then back on your heels to sense where your center is.
2. Think of your head as floating on the top of your spine, not sinking down into your neck, and gently allow the head to lift and lengthen the entire spine.
3. Keep your chin parallel to the floor, not up or down, otherwise you'll constrict the top vertebrae.
4. Let your shoulders release down; don't let them inch up to your ears, as we tend to do when tense. And let your arms dangle to the sides.

5. Hold your stomach in firmly, but do it with your muscles; don't hold your breath or squeeze the buttocks.
6. The buttocks should be held firmly but not clenched, and should line up with your back and legs, not jutting out. You may have to tuck your buttocks and pelvis under first in an exaggerated way and then slowly release until you get into position.
7. Now think of lengthening the spine—imagine putting a pocket of air between all the vertebrae so they all float and lift. And at the same time think of widening the back—just let your shoulders release outward and fill your lungs.

Do not push, on any of these steps. Pushing and pulling only tighten muscles and prevent you from achieving that relaxed posture that will ward off aches and pains later on.

As you walk, visualize yourself lengthening and widening and relaxing any muscles not in use at the moment. Instead of pounding each foot into the street, think of pushing off with the ball of the foot and then letting go in the hip joints so the leg swings gently out in a smooth, controlled, but relaxed movement. Let the arms swing naturally in opposition to the foot (right arm swings forward with left leg).

As you sit, relax but don't release into a slump. Keep your back straight—that's easiest to do when you press your back firmly into the back of the chair while keeping your feet planted on the floor. (Short people should get a pillow to put at the small of the back in order to keep the feet on the floor).

Now whenever you think of it, wherever you are, stand up straight.

Other I-Hate-to-Move Tricks

These are little games you can play with yourself to encourage habits that will get you moving.

1. Get off the bus or subway train one stop before your destination—whether it's on the way to work, the store, or home.
2. When you've mastered that, make it two stops.
3. Run all errands within a couple of miles by walking.
4. While doing chores, be very conscious of your posture and make sure your stomach is pulled in and your back is straight at all times.
5. Do household chores in rapid succession, with no break in between, to get your pulse up and keep it up. Why bother jogging when the carpet needs vacuuming and the tub needs scrubbing?

6. Cultivate a fear of elevators and always take the stairs.
7. Never wear tight clothes that restrict your natural movement, whether at work or at home. It's hard enough to get enthusiastic about moving without having your clothes inhibit you before you even start.
8. Get to a mirror whenever you dress and undress—the naked picture tells you where you need improving—and where the improvement has already begun.
9. Never phone any neighbor within half a block of home or five floors of an office. Let your legs, not your fingers, do the walking.
10. Imagine that there is a television camera focused on you at all times throughout the day. That will remind you to sit up straight and make every movement graceful and energetic.

I-HATE-TO-EXERCISE CALORIE-BURNING CHART

Activity	Calories Burned per Hour
Lying down	80
Sitting	100
Standing up	140
Driving a car	120

However, if you try some of the above exercises while you sit, stand, or lie down, you can easily double the number of calories you will burn.

12
Learning to Love Stress

Coping With the Stress of Life

STRESS ALONE WILL NOT KILL—if you learn how to handle it. Coping does not mean coddling yourself so you avoid stress. Quite the contrary. There are techniques that actually help you face more intense pressure than you could before, confidently, successfully, and safely.

Once you can recognize the early-warning symptoms of stress and master the simple techniques, you can turn off the stress alarm before it starts doing you harm. You can handle pressure and tension smoothly, without wasting energy, and then dive back into the fray with greater chances for success at whatever you do. Each new, small victory serves as a healing tonic to the body and renders you that much better equipped to handle the next difficulty expertly. It is a subtle, cyclical process that allows you to make stress work for you in your life. And it all begins when you learn how to relax your mind and body.

Easy to say. Now here's how to do it.

Recognize the Early Warning Signs of Stress

These symptoms are your body's way of telling you to ease up—if only for a minute—because you're reaching stress overload. None of these symptoms is particularly harmful in itself, but if you ignore them, you could be headed for trouble.

1. Sweaty hands or cold hands, especially if one hand is colder than the other.
2. Shortness of breath.
3. Being susceptible to every cold or virus that goes around (because the physical strains of distress have lowered your immunity).
4. Headaches, tiredness, irritability.
5. Indigestion, diarrhea, too frequent urination.
6. Muscle spasms or a tightness in the jaw, back of the neck, shoulders, or lower back.
7. Difficulty sleeping, or sleeping too much without feeling rested.
8. Finding yourself increasing your eating, drinking, smoking, or use of drugs.
9. Moodiness and difficulty concentrating. .
10. Becoming suddenly accident-prone.

As soon as you notice one of these warning signs, stop whatever you're doing, and try one of the stress-management techniques described below.

Ten-Second Stress Fix

You can do this discreetly anytime, anywhere. The technique combines elements of self-hypnosis, meditation, and relaxation therapy. You remain alert but relaxed, able to give yourself suggestions and follow through with them. If you use it throughout the day at the first signs of tension or pressure, you should be able to prevent the whole cycle of the stress response from escalating into bad stress. Instead of squandering your energy on nervous tension, you will be better equipped to focus your energy on the task at hand.

In addition to relieving stress and controlling your energy, the elements of self-hypnosis incorporated within the exercise can be helpful in changing habits—the stress fix can reinforce your willpower to follow through on changes when you feel a moment of relapse approaching. The stress fix keeps you in control.

With this technique, as with self-hypnosis or the learning of any new skill, the more you do it and become familiar with how it feels to be deeply relaxed, the faster you will be able to sink into relaxation. You'll know you've really mastered this approach when you can rename it the Three-Second Stress Fix.

Here are the steps.

1. *Squeeze your thumb and index finger together hard for two seconds, at the moment when you're feeling acutely tense (or at any point when you feel the impulse to engage in a habit you want to change or simply when you need a peaceful break.)*

   This squeezing cue serves two functions. First, if you squeeze hard (you can even use your fingernail into your thumb), the tensing of those muscles in your hand and arm and the slight discomfort of the pressure will give you a controlled physical outlet for the frustration that stressful emotions arouse. And second, it will transfer your attention and your tension and mental pain from the issue at hand to your fingers.

2. *Now, roll your eyes heavenward as you inhale deeply for two more seconds—still squeezing the fingers.*

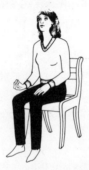

   You can think of this as rolling your eyes in mock disgust and wonder at the events in life that can drive you to feel this tense. It helps if you allow it to feel like an almost comical gesture—if you can make fun of a situation or, better yet, yourself and your overreaction to a situation, you feel in control and ultimately on top of it—in short, you stop feeling stressed by it.

   The roll of the eyes, however, should not be a movement from side to side as much as a sweep from your chest upward to your forehead and beyond as if you were trying to see through a skylight on the top of your head. Close your eyes at the end of the sweep, though keep facing skyward. If someone else were watching, the last visible bit before you closed your lids would be the whites of your eyes.

3. *Hold your breath for 2 seconds while still gazing upward beneath closed eyes. Continue looking up even though your eyes may open very slightly and flutter.*

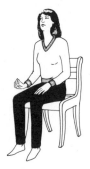

4. *Then exhale, slowly, completely, letting your fingers, your eyes, and all the tension in your body go—take 4 seconds.*

As you feel the pleasant release of tension from your fingers it will be the cue to your jaw, head, shoulders, and your entire body to go pleasantly slack. It helps to listen to the steady whooshing sound you make as you exhale and imagine the tension as rushing water flowing out of every limb. You may find as you exhale that it helps to repeat silently words like "peace" or "let it go" or "it's only life," that you will also use in the relaxation exercises described next.

If you have more than ten seconds, you can use this stress fix as the lead-in to a longer session. After reaching stage 4, you can give yourself suggestions about changing habits or feelings. The brain is especially responsive to such suggestions in this relaxed (trancelike) state. You can say things like: "When I open my eyes, I will not be hungry and when I do get hungry I will have a yearning for a nice, fresh carrot"; or "I will feel calm and relaxed even if the kids yell and the dogs bark—I will feel warm and happy they're alive and healthy."

Whatever suggestions you give yourself during the extended session, it helps to end with something like the following: "When I open my eyes I will feel relaxed, refreshed, alert, and happy. I will open my eyes on the count of three: one . . . two . . . three."

The Invisible Quick Fix

Once you become comfortable with the ten-second procedure, you will not only be able to do that version more quickly, but you will also be able to get nearly as much tension relief with an abbreviated version that does not even involve closing your eyes and thus can be done in full view, without any overt sign that you are doing anything more unusual than breathing. The shorter version works only if you have done the original stress fix long enough that your brain instantly connects the finger-squeezing cue with deep relaxation. A few weeks of steady practice should be all you need.

The quick fix is an especially handy technique to use right before delivering a speech or during a tense meeting or any time you are in the heat of battle and need to calm down but stay alert.

1. Just squeeze your thumb and finger together as in the longer version, keeping your hand in your pocket or under the conference table. Take a deep breath and hold a fraction of a second.
2. Then release the fingers and exhale slowly but quietly.

Using both versions of the stress fix should enable you to return to your task with renewed strength and patience. As soon as you find yourself slipping into anger or anxiety again, do the stress fix all over. A few seconds of strategic stress release can save you hours of frustration later, and, in a lifetime, perhaps years of wear and tear.

End the I-Hate-to-Wait Stress Blues

Everyone—no matter how high or low—has to wait for something, usually at dozens of points in every day. Whether you're waiting for the bus or the chauffeur, time is passing and you don't like it. But some of us are worse about it than others. And most of us inflict more pain and suffering on ourselves at those times than we need to.

If you hate to wait, if the sight of a line at a place you're about to enter makes your heart sink and your blood boil, welcome to the club. However, if you have any interest in the survival of the club's membership, probably the single-most important lesson you can learn—after the Ten-Second Stress Fix—is mastering how to wait without stress.

This strategy will not make you love lines—the instructions here are for stress reduction not frontal lobotomy—but it will enable you, when you find yourself in line, and you will, to pass the time calmly and constructively.

1. Recognize the stress signs.
    Are your hands clenched, are you glancing at your watch impatiently every five seconds? Are you saying to yourself something

like, "How can I be so stupid? I should have known there would be a line and left enough time. And just look at how long that other idiot is taking. There's no way I can make it on time now."

What's the point? Nobody else is going to let you butt ahead because everybody else is fuming, too. And nobody cares that you're too important and busy to be kept standing around like this because all of them, from the bag lady to the gent with the fedora, think the same of themselves. And if you're going to be late and have to suffer later, why torture yourself now? Try the following steps instead.

2. Take a deep breath, and use this time to practice the stress fix.

You can do the longer ten-second version, eyes closed and all. Everyone is so busy working up to ulcers and heart conditions that no one will notice.

3. Expect to wait at some point every day and prepare yourself.

If you can't have a book with you at all times, at least keep a poem in your wallet that you'd like to memorize for when you're washed ashore on a desert island with only the literature in your brain to amuse you. If you've already memorized the poem in an earlier waiting session, and you haven't picked a new one yet, recite the old poem to yourself.

4. If you haven't come equipped with literary props, use the time to see the funny side of humanity.

Seek out the amusing aspect of everything around you; notice how silly other people look as they stand in line and stew. Scrutinize strangers' faces and make up stories about who they are, what they do, how their love life is going, how long they have to live, as if you were a novelist and these were your characters.

Or socialize—if there is someone appealing next to you, strike up a conversation. It will certainly make the time pass pleasantly, and you never know where these things will lead.

5. Exercise while you wait.

As you'll see if you turn back to chapter 11, "I-Hate-to-Exercise Exercises," there are any number of discreet movements you can do to strengthen muscles. Several that you can do without drawing attention to yourself are: head rolls, shoulder lifts, waist twists, small knee bends, ankle circles, standing up straight with stomach pulled in tight, lifting up onto the balls of the feet and balancing, buttocks tucks (if you're wearing a coat). If you don't mind what others think, there is no reason why you can't use the time to run in place, or jump up and down to get your blood moving.

You know you've got the I-hate-to-wait stress licked when you find yourself mildly disappointed at the end of a day in which your new waiting skills have not been put to the test.

Peace Plan—Ten-Minute Relaxation Technique

You should allow at least 10 minutes for this exercise; if you have more time, it works even better.

P Position must be comfortable.
E Environment must be quiet, no interruptions.
A Attitude must be passive; let everything go.
C Catchword or catchphrase, such as "Peace" or "Relax" or "Let the tension go," helps.
E Elation will follow.

Position. The most comfortable positions are usually either lying down on your back or sitting on a cushioned chair that supports the back, lets your feet rest flat on the floor, and your hands settle (palms slightly up) on the arms of the chair or on your thighs.

Environment. Take the phones off the hook, close the door, and let everyone in the household know that you do not want to be interrupted unless the firemen are at the door with the hoses.

Attitude. Don't test yourself or try to rate how deeply you relaxed this time as opposed to last on a scale of 1 to 10. No matter what happens, you will always emerge more relaxed than you began, so let yourself drift and see where relaxation takes you.

As you breathe in and out deeply and regularly, focus your attention up and down your body, looking for any little pockets of tension and let them go.

Release the tightness in your jaw and neck muscles, where most people concentrate their tension without even realizing it, by letting your jaw drop open and your head gently flop down. Let your neck lengthen as your shoulders sink down several inches; your chest should merely obey the smooth billows of your breath. The stomach will slacken—let it. As the muscles in the thighs and calves release, allow your legs to flop open (a position of relaxed vulnerability that women, especially, often feel quite self-conscious about at first—that's why you must have a private, protected environment). Feel your toes uncurl and your feet sink heavily into the floor.

Sometimes you'll find that as the tension escapes from your mind and body, all the worries of the day seem to rush in to fill the vacuum. Don't panic. Try examining a few of those problems to see if they look less formidable in this calmer state of mind.

Or if you don't want to spend your relaxation time rehashing worries, then think of your brain as a movie screen with a bad movie playing and either turn off the lights and make the screen go dark or speed to the end of the reel and make the screen go bright white, whichever you find easier to do—people vary. You may have to try wiping the slate clean repeatedly, as worries can often be persistent little nags.

Catchword. Repeating the catchword in a rhythmic drone helps you wipe the screen clean, blocking out extraneous thoughts as well as background noises much the way white sound works. It is hypnotic and helps gently nudge away troubles.

If no word or phrase comes to you right away, you may find simply focusing intently on the rhythmic whooshing sound of your own breathing is relaxing, and counting with each breath helps you pace your breathing—"Inhale one, two, three; exhale one, two, three."

Expect Elation. Expect to feel better after 10, even 5 minutes of this therapy—20 minutes feels as good as a nap. Before you end the session and before you open your eyes again, say to yourself quite explicitly, "I will open my eyes and feel relaxed, refreshed, cheerful, and ready to face the world." You might also want to give yourself a specific suggestion about something you might want to do next; for example, "I will feel relaxed, refreshed, and ready to tackle studying for that test."

And you will.

Muscle Relaxation for Sleep, Headaches, and All Stress-Related Disorders

The aim. To get rid of the tension in your whole body by tightening and then relaxing the muscles from head to toe.

At first you will work each muscle group twice. After practice, you may not need this repetition. Concentrate on how each part feels when tensed and savor the warmth of release. The concentration will release your mind; the tightening and relaxing will teach you how to release the body and ease the aches and pains that tightness brings. When you finish, you will either get up again thoroughly relaxed or simply slip into sleep.

BEGIN WITH A BREATH

1. Sit down or lie down and get comfortable. Now inhale deeply, feeling first your chest, then the rib cage, and then the abdomen fill; hold 5 seconds. Exhale slowly, feeling your abdomen, your rib cage, and then your chest sink down and relax. Repeat 3 times.

HEAD

1. Roll your head gently from side to side as if saying no, then up and down as if saying yes. You're loosened up and ready to begin.
2. Raise your eyebrows high to tense your forehead, and hold for 5 seconds. Release, take a breath, and feel the forehead relax. Repeat.
3. Close your eyes tightly, hold 5 seconds. Release. Repeat.
4. Wrinkle your nose and cheeks and smile tightly, hold 5 seconds. Release. Repeat.
5. Jut your jaw, then open your mouth wide, hold. Release. Repeat.
6. Blow your cheeks open as if they were balloons, hold. Release. Repeat.
   Now take a breath and feel how relaxed your whole head feels.

NECK AND SHOULDERS

1. Lift your chin as high as you can while you look up to the ceiling and over to the wall behind you, hold. Release. Repeat.
2. Touch your chin to your chest to tighten the back of the neck and shoulders (don't let your shoulders hunch), hold. Release. Repeat.
3. Lift your shoulders to your ears, hold. Release. Repeat.
4. Push your shoulders forward as if you would have them touch in front of you, hold. Release. Repeat.
5. Pull your shoulders back and down on the bed or floor as if you were trying to make them touch behind you, hold. Release. Repeat.

Take a deep breath and notice again how relaxed your head, neck, and shoulders now feel.

ARMS

1. Stretch your right arm out as long as possible, reaching right through the fingertips; clench and unclench your fist twice. Release. Repeat.
2. Stretch your left arm out as long as possible, reaching through the fingertips; clench and unclench your fist twice. Release. Repeat.

CHEST AND ABDOMEN

1. Inhale deeply and fill the chest, rib cage, and abdomen, hold. Exhale, letting first the abdomen, then the rib cage, and finally the chest relax. Repeat.
2. Tighten the abdomen, pulling it down toward your back (but don't tighten the buttocks, yet), hold. Release. Repeat.

BUTTOCKS, THIGHS, AND LEGS

1. Squeeze the buttocks, hold. Release. Repeat.
2. Concentrate on your upper right thigh, tighten, hold. Release. Repeat.
3. Flex your right foot and straighten your entire leg, focusing on tensing the calf this time; point your toes, then flex again. Release. Repeat.
4. Concentrate on your upper left thigh, tighten, hold. Release. Repeat.
5. Flex your left foot and straighten the leg, focusing on tensing the calf; then point your toes, flex again. Release. Repeat.

Now feel how heavy and relaxed your whole body feels. If any spots still feel tense, go over them again.

Then breathe deeply and slowly 3 times, sinking deeper with each breath into a comforting, quieting relaxed state.

Talk Nicely to Yourself

Imagine, if you will, an ordinary stressful situation. You have a deadline for a report to the boss, you're afraid you won't finish on time, your hands are sweating, and your heart is thumping so loud you can't concentrate.

Now what is that little voice inside you saying?

What little voice, you say? You may not even be conscious of it, but all of us talk to ourselves. A little internal commentator is constantly assessing the environment and reporting on how we're doing: "This looks threatening—I don't think I can handle it, at least not without a cigarette."

The voice can be calming. But for most of us, it is not nearly as encouraging as it could be. All too often we find ourselves saying things like: "I'll never make it. Why did I wait so long to start this project? I'd better hurry up, just get moving, but how? If I mess this up, I'll probably never get that promotion. Boy, I hate this job; I hate my boss. I hate myself for getting so worked up. I give up."

Blood pressure rises, arteries begin to clog—and all for what? It doesn't get the work done; in fact it interferes with efficiency. And it surely isn't a pleasant way to pass the time.

So what can you do instead?

Practice talking nicely. Be better company to yourself. Encourage yourself.

Be on the lookout for negative, self-defeating words. As soon as you hear yourself uttering "must," "should," "ought," "can't," "never," you know you're simply escalating the anxiety.

Here's an example of the kind of negative perspective that promotes stress—Stress Talk—and the more positive alternatives you could adopt to help reduce stress—Stressless Talk.

Stress Talk	*Stressless Talk*
I'll never get this done	Just dive in and take it one step at a time
I'm so nervous I can't think straight	Take a deep breath, relax, and let's get started. Once I get rolling I know I'll feel and work better
What if they hate what I come up with even if I can do it in time?	You never can tell what they'll think, but things have worked out before, they probably will again. I'll just do the best I can
I never should have waited so long to start; why do I always do this to myself?	Everybody would feel some tension in a situation like this. I can handle it. Come on brain, use that adrenaline and let's get this job done. I think I'll treat myself to something special when this is all over

Next time you find yourself in a situation that is making you feel anxious and tense, try to listen to what your inner voice is saying. Write it down. You'll see how pointless and self-defeating it can be. Then write down a more soothing alternative. It shouldn't be mindless pep talk of the "Hey, kid, you're the greatest no matter what happens and besides it's not the end of the world" variety. It has to be something you can hear yourself saying and believe; it should be realistic, but encouraging. It should also be simple. The truth is that whatever is causing you distress is not likely to end the world, or even your life. So put the fears and anxieties in perspective, calm yourself down, and then you can tackle the real problem at hand.

Once you've written down some Stressless alternatives to Stress Talk, use them when you feel the pressure building. Every time you hear yourself chiseling away at your confidence with that negative little voice, change the script. You'll feel better and cope better.

Daydream, Visualize, Rehearse Events

Daydreaming. This is not a waste of time. You can make excellent use of your visualizing powers to prepare yourself in advance to face a stress-provoking situation.

Daydream about something that makes you nervous, visualize it in complete detail, rehearse what you would do. If you want to ask for a raise, go through what you will say and all the possible things that your adversary might say. If you want to ask for a date, do the same. Then when you go through the experience, it will seem familiar, comfortable, like an old shoe, and you will feel much more confident about handling it.

Visualization. An excellent training technique. Professional athletes use visualization to augment their physical training. You not only learn a sport or a new movement by seeing yourself do it in your mind's eye and then practicing it until it feels right, but you can also enhance your practice by relaxing and visualizing your body moving as it should—it trains your brain to coordinate.,

Visualization is also being used to fight disease (as described in chapter 2). In this therapy, people picture their white blood cells and lymphocytes destroying invading cancer cells, blowing up tumors. Such visualization actually seems to energize the immune system, encouraging it to behave in the way we imagine.

In the same way, visualization can serve to reduce stress. For example, if you are prone to anger and hostility, you can visualize yourself in a situation that typically makes you angry. Then visualize yourself—in vivid detail—responding calmly instead: follow what you'd say, how you'd move, even imagine how calm you'd feel. This rehearsal prepares you to carry out your plan, because when the situation presents itself, you've actually already been through it and reacted the way you want to—calmly and fully in control.

Rehearse. Follow these steps:

1. You are driving in your car with the world's slowest driver blocking the lane ahead.

   Imagine getting angry and banging the steering wheel, shouting expletives, and behaving boorishly.

   Now picture yourself in the driver's seat, saying, "I wish that car would speed up, but there's nothing I can do, so I may as well look at the scenery or listen to the radio." Go on to imagine how calm and unhurried you feel as you take in sights along the road you never had the time to notice before.

2. You lose your job.

   Imagine the worst and go through exactly what you would do, how you would feel. If the fear is going to haunt you, and make you nervous every time a difficult task or confrontation comes up at work, then you should at least know concretely what you might face. It will help you make plans if the worst should actually come to pass, and it may help you to see that it may not be such a frightening prospect after all.

3. You lose the love of your spouse, your children.

   This exercise may help you see how important these elements of your life are and may help you get your priorities straight. Then you can order your actions, your time appropriately, something that always reduces feelings of stress.

4. Now you pick a scene that typically makes you angry or anxious or fearful. Picture your usual reaction. Then repeat the scene all over, this time reacting the way you would like to. Go through it in full detail, as an actor playing a scene. Eventually you will be able to direct your real-life actions as fully as you directed your daydreams.

Laugh or Cry—The Healthiest of Exercises

Don't hold back. Let the laughter and the tears rip—they may just be the oldest and pleasantest stress-relief known to humankind.

We all have experienced at one time or another that limp-muscled feeling after a good laugh or cry when you feel drained, relaxed, and thoroughly refreshed. Scientific research is beginning to show that this sensation stems from more than simple muscle relaxation after a laughing or crying workout—though that does play a part. There are also biochemical changes taking place that seem to defuse stress.

Tears triggered by emotions contain a higher concentration of proteins than those triggered by irritation, according to a Minnesota researcher. And they may actually carry away from the body the harmful chemical by-products of stress. Laughter, too, seems to trigger the release of endorphins (the body's natural euphoric) and other chemicals which not only make us feel terrific but may reverse some of the damages of distress.

Here are some pointers on how to encourage laughter and tears.

1. Make it a point to have on your bookshelf a couple of works that never fail to make you laugh out loud. (Books by P. G. Wodehouse, E. B. White, James Thurber, Damon Runyon, and Mark Twain are pretty good bets.) If there are any amusing plays or movies being shown in town, indulge yourself. (The same goes for books or movies that can move you to tears.)
2. Try occasionally to look at even your most frightening problems with a distant observer's eye, seeking out like a detective, the smallest element that could be seen as amusing, silly, downright hilarious. Comedians get paid to make us laugh at a painful experience. While we cannot all be comics, we can remind ourselves to try to view even the most serious events with a comical eye. Once you can laugh, the pain and the anxiety usually diminish.
3. Give yourself and others permission to cry. When your children or your friends begin to sob, don't say, "There, there, don't cry." And especially avoid telling little boys that "Big boys don't cry." They should. It is probably no coincidence that men, who are discouraged from crying in our society, suffer a larger share of heart disease and other stress-related disorders than do women. We all need a good cry now and then. Be sympathetic, but let the tears flow.
4. Once you start crying, give it all you've got. Don't hold back. And don't feel as though you have to stick to the subject. You may as well dredge up some recent hurts that you would have liked to cry about but didn't have the chance. Cry until you can laugh. Laugh until you cry. You'll feel wonderful afterward.

Do-It-Yourself Massage

Massage nearly always rubs you the right way. Some masseurs claim that an hour of massage is the equivalent of two hours of sleep. One thing is certain: it feels wonderful, relaxes tight muscles, and makes you feel refreshed.

Massage, like making love, is hard to do alone, but not impossible. There are a number of things you can do to relieve your own tension. And you can do these anywhere, sitting at your desk, in front of the television, or in the bath.

D-I-Y FACE AND SCALP MASSAGE

Lie down. Cover your face with your hands and rest in the darkness a moment. Then use your fingertips and thumbs in stroking circular motions beginning at the forehead, sweeping down to the temples, along the cheeks, jaw, and the bridge of the nose. Fan out along the scalp with continued pressure and circular motions, pausing at the tender points above the ears and at the base of the scalp where tense muscles tend to knot up.

D-I-Y NECK AND SHOULDERS MASSAGE

Reach your fingers up over your shoulders and as far down your back as you can, pressing the fingertips hard on either side of the spine. Squeeze and knead as strongly as you can, moving outward from the spine and upward to the shoulders. Use your right hand to knead the left shoulder and vice versa. Then use both hands as you move up along the neck to the base of the scalp.

D-I-Y FOOT MASSAGE

Chinese medicine subscribes to the belief that every nerve ending in the body and every organ has a link to some part of the foot. Massaging the feet, they would argue, is like massaging the whole body. For those who have had a foot massage, there can be little doubt that the Chinese are on to something. Despite the daily abuse our feet take, they remain highly sensitive and receptive to massage. And they are one of the easiest parts of the body to massage by yourself.

It is best to soak the feet for a few minutes before you begin.

Then sit down and rest your left ankle on the right knee. Make a fist with your right hand, steadying the foot with your left hand, and knead the sole with your knuckles moving in circles.

Hold the foot in both hands and vigorously work over the entire foot using thumbs and fingertips.

Next, on the top of the foot, run your thumb along the valleys between the bones from toes to ankle.

Squeeze the whole foot, pressing the heels of your hands into the sole and fanning out to the edges.

Grasp each toe and gently pull and twist; don't forget the spaces between the toes.

Slap the soles and sides of the foot gently; rotate the ankles.

Finish by placing one hand on top of the foot, the other underneath, and holding your hands still.

Repeat for the other foot.

Now relax.

Antistress Diet

The strain of stress increases your need for all vitamins and minerals, especially the B-complex and C vitamins. Vitamin C is critical to the functioning of the adrenal glands, and the B vitamins promote the health of the nervous system—both crucial in handling stress.

High-potency vitamins—often labeled stress vitamins—usually have much higher doses than you need, and all you wind up with is vitamin-packed, canary-yellow urine. Vitamins B and C are water soluble, and whatever our bodies do not make immediate use of simply passes through the system into the toilet.

If you're feeling under acute stress, it probably cannot hurt to take an extra multivitamin or even one of the stress formulas that have moderate levels of B and C vitamins

But the best thing you can do under stress is to eat more citrus fruits and fish, chicken, green vegetables, and whole grains, which are rich in the C and B-complex vitamins.

Also bear in mind that stress can raise cholesterol levels. So it is an especially good time to try to cut back on foods high in cholesterol and fat—meat, eggs, butter, cream.

Cakes, cookies, and ice cream, which often seem soothing in times of stress, can ultimately make you feel worse. The high sugar content may make your blood-sugar levels roller-coaster and your mood follow suit. There is enough strain on your body in adapting to the changes that stress brings without having to adapt to dramatic changes in blood-sugar levels as well. In addition, these dessert foods are also usually high in fats. (See chapter 15 for more tips on how to cut back on cholesterol and fat.)

Similarly, though being under stress may make you want to reach for a cigarette or a drink, these may only aggravate your tension. And they will increase your feelings of being out of control—which is exactly what triggered the stress response in the first place and the feeling that will keep you under stress without relief.

Eat citrus fruits, vegetables, fish, chicken, and whole grains.

Avoid caffeine, alcohol; fatty, cholesterol-rich foods like meat and eggs and butter, as well as sweets.

Antistress Exercises

Anything that gets you moving—the more vigorously the better—takes your mind off your troubles, increases your endorphin levels, and makes you feel relaxed and renewed afterward. (See more detailed discussion of what exercise does to benefit your heart, lungs, bones, and brain in chapter 10.)

1. If you start steaming about some troubles at work or at home, get up immediately—before you say anything you'll regret—and take a brisk walk around the block. You will return with a clearer head and greater patience to cope.
2. Incorporate exercise into your weekly schedule. Having a regular, dependable escape valve keeps tension from building up to explosive levels. And it enables you to work harder and more efficiently if you are assured of a set time and place where you will be able to let all the tension go.
3. Do small limbering and stretching movements throughout the day, at your desk, as you walk to lunch, as you talk on the phone (see chapter 11 for suggestions). Like the Ten-Second Stress Fix, these quickie stretches will keep muscles from getting so knotted up that your best efforts cannot help you unwind at the end of the day.
4. Pick an exercise that is sufficiently challenging and demanding to occupy your mind as well as your body. If worries seem to plague you, then perhaps running is not the first activity to try, as you may not be able to get the problems out of your head. A sport requiring the acquisition of a new skill—dance or racquet ball or skating—demands full concentration and often provides more relief for your mind and body.

Sing a Song for Sagging Spirits

When you feel very tense or depressed, raise your voice in song and you'll find it actually helps calm you down and lift your spirits as well.

You have to take deep, regular breaths to sing and that same regular breathing has a calming effect. You have to loosen your throat and neck muscles to keep the voice from sounding pinched, and that, too, tends to exert a soothing influence. Concentrating on the rhythm, the tune, and the words distracts you from whatever is troubling you—so that even if the song is the blues, it will be cheerier than focusing on your own blues. If you feel self-conscious about singing out at the top of your lungs, get in the shower and belt it out. There isn't a much healthier way to drown your sorrows.

13
Change Your Type A Ways

How to Stop Being Type A and Start Being Healthy

SO YOU THINK you're Type A, eh?

Find out whether you are, to what degree you are (most of us have a mixture of Type A and Type B traits), and which aspects of your behavior really put you at the most risk for heart disease and stroke, not to mention ulcers, headaches, backaches, and a host of other ailments affected by the chronic stress of the Type A response to life.

Test Yourself—Are You Type A?

Pinning down whether you are a Type A person is a tricky task. Sometimes Type A's are the last to know—they often do not recognize many of their own traits, gestures, and facial grimaces, all of which can be telltale clues.

So, in addition to taking this test, you might want to get someone you trust and can be open with to go over the list of Type A and Type B characteristics following the test to see if they recognize some of the behavioral signs that you might miss by yourself.

Score as follows:

4 If you agree strongly or the statement nearly always applies to you.
3 If you agree mildly or it applies often.
2 If you agree sometimes or it applies sometimes.
1 If you disagree or it applies rarely.
0 If you disagree strongly or it almost never applies.

1. I am extremely competitive, and I suspect that people who don't seem competitive are just disguising their true impulses.
2. When I get angry, I feel like hauling off and socking someone.
3. Most people in the world would stretch the truth if it helped them step up the success ladder.
4. I wish there were more hours in the day to get everything done, but then I guess I'd just schedule more things to do.
5. I hate waiting in line, and I get really antsy when other people take a long time to make their point in a discussion.
6. I have trouble getting along with my supervisors.
7. I play to win at work and at sports—otherwise why bother?
8. I push myself harder than most people; I walk fast, talk fast, and constantly strive to do more in less time.
9. I need deadlines to get things accomplished so even when someone else hasn't set deadlines I set them up for myself to keep me moving at a fast clip.
10. I find it quite hard to relax; no matter how long my vacations are, I never quite fully unwind before it's time to get back to work.

YOUR SCORE

Extremely Type A—33–40.
Strongly Type A—25–32.
Tending toward Type A—11–24.
Basically Type B—0–10.

How to Spot Type A Behavior in Others

- They're competitive, aggressive, impatient, always feeling a sense of time passing too quickly to get everything done they've scheduled.
- When they talk, they often pound their fists into their hands, clench their teeth, or repeat other nervous gestures. (Grinding teeth at night is another telltale sign.)
- They often impatiently finish other people's sentences or interject "yes, yes, yes" or "uh-huh, uh-huh" to hurry the speaker on.
- They always move, eat, and walk rapidly.
- They can't stand waiting in line or getting stuck in a traffic lane behind someone slow.
- They become readily angry, hostile, and frustrated when things don't go their way.

- They find it genuinely difficult to listen to others and always feel compelled to bring the conversation around to a topic that interests them.
- They try to do several things at once—reading while shaving, dictating letters while driving.
- They feel guilty when they relax.
- They are not necessarily the executives or the big shots; anyone can be a Type A. In fact, top executives may be less vulnerable to Type A behavior and heart disease than various underlings.

How to Spot Type B Behavior in Others

- Type Bs are more aware and confident of their capabilities, able to accept their own inadequacies.
- They rarely feel that sense of time urgency and impatience that haunts the Type A.
- They are not terribly hostile and do not feel compelled to discuss their accomplishments except when the situation demands it.
- They have drive and can work and play competitively, but they do it more for the satisfaction and pleasure than to prove their superiority to all others.
- They can work without needing to feel wound up and agitated.
- They can relax, go on vacation, and really enjoy it without guilt.

Type A Children

Even young children can begin manifesting many of these personality traits. Often, their characteristics are not yet full blown versions of the adult. So keep on the lookout for subtler signs:

- They are always ready to go on an outing before the rest of the family, and they get very impatient waiting for the family to pull together.
- They become anxious if they're not always at least 15 minutes early for school or any other activity.
- They become easily angry and upset—with others and themselves—if they don't catch on fast enough to a new physical or intellectual skill.
- They focus so intently on competing and winning, no matter what they're doing, that they don't seem able to enjoy the activity itself.

Steps Toward Changing Your Type A Ways

Type A behavior patterns are themselves a serious set of warning signals. But for once, treating the symptoms actually treats the disease. Again, these traits are not immutable. They are largely learned behavior and can be "unlearned" too. (Read chapter 6, "Heart Disease," for more about Type A behavior.)

Changing Type A behavior now could save your life. Severely Type A men who have already had one heart attack and who then modify just a few of their obvious Type A habits have been shown in studies to be able to halve their risk for a second coronary event. Changing now to ward off the first heart attack is even wiser and healthier.

Modifying behavior can unquestionably reduce the excessive and inappropriate secretions of the stress hormones (especially epinephrine and norepinephrine) that are thought to do the damage to Type A's. While certain drugs being tested may prove helpful in blocking the effects of stress hormones and even in changing Type A reactions under stress (see discussion of beta blockers in chapter 6), for now the most powerful tool within our control is our behavior.

Remember, you will not be able to transform yourself from a Type A to a Type B. But who wants to? Some aspects of Type A behavior aren't all that bad; they can be quite productive. But the key is learning which traits help us and which do not. Making small changes—but the right ones—and learning new stress-management techniques (see chapter 12) can make the difference not only between life and death but also between enjoying life and just passing through in a hurry.

Don't expect the externals in your life to change dramatically. You'll probably work the same hours, toil with equally intense drive, and continue to be successful. The major change will be subtler—your mood will be better, your attitude about life will become more tolerant. Your efficiency should improve along with your health. You'll probably feel fewer aches and pains, get fewer colds. Don't expect other people to notice right away. But then again, don't be surprised if they do.

The following techniques will help you modify a number of small daily habits and attitudes. Each change may seem insignificant in itself. But it is not. Each time you relax instead of getting angry, each time you laugh instead of fume, you are saving your body wear and tear. These good effects build up like a savings account (just as the damaging effects, if you don't change your old ways, accumulate like a bad debt). One deep breath instead of a shouted curse, ten times a day, seven days a week, starts adding up to some impressive bodily savings by the end of a year or two. With interest—added interest in life.

You can't lose.

Changing Type A Behavior

1. Stop being proud of being Type A.

   It is not the Purple Heart of corporate life; it is not to be confused with being "typed" as an "A student," much as the words sound similar; it is not proof that you are a hard worker and an important person.

   If you've been successful at work, it is in spite of your Type A leanings, which are often hostile and irrational, not because of them. There are actually more calm Type Bs in the highest-level positions; Type A's are more likely to end up in middle management. Type A's may work hard, but so can Type Bs, without wasting energy on being angry, hostile, and overly rushed all the time.

2. Set realistic goals concerning which aspects of your personality you can change and how long it will take.

   There is no virtue in setting your sights on achievements you can never attain and then chastising yourself or pushing harder when you seem to be falling short. It's not "compromising" or "settling for less" to be realistic, and it makes life generally, and living with yourself specifically, a great deal more relaxed and enjoyable.

3. Make a contract with yourself for each goal, write it down, and work on one modification at a time.

   Make your goal very specific. "I will not eat alone for the next week. I will not stamp my foot and fume while waiting in line for the next two weeks." No abstracts. Keep a daily record of how you're doing.

4. Hurry sickness is half the problem; you have to find ways to slow down.

   • Wake up 20 minutes earlier so you can have more time to get ready in the mornings—time to dress, eat breakfast, and travel to work, even if there's a ridiculous traffic jam. You don't want to start the day feeling rushed.

   • Schedule into each day 20 minutes of uninterrupted relaxation time alone—don't just hope you'll catch a few minutes here and there.

5. Don't schedule more than you really have time for.

If you get through your paces early, don't schedule more. Take off some time to cultivate the calmer pleasures of a slow-paced meal out or a leisurely stroll in the park.

6. Take off your watch.

You may be late now and then, and it may make you more nervous at first not knowing the time, but eventually it will keep you from getting that unnecessary burst of epinephrine (adrenaline) that Type A's often get dozens of times a day, whenever they glance down at their watch to see a concrete reminder of time passing.

7. Plan one event every week that puts friendship above business or that encourages you to laugh or feel playful.

A semibusiness lunch doesn't count. Pack a sandwich, take it to the zoo, and eat it while sitting in front of the gorilla cage. Catch a movie at lunchtime that makes you laugh. Come up with one funny story or joke a week, and tell it to your friends.

8. Start a regular exercise routine.

It doesn't have to be rigorous or lengthy at first. But you should schedule a regular time, three days a week—all right, you can start out just on weekends—for some specific activity. A brisk walk, a warm-up and cool-down routine with a bout of jumping rope in between. It doesn't matter what the exercise is in the beginning. But it will help get rid of anger, relieve stress, make you feel more cheerful and better able to handle pressures calmly and competently. (See chapter 10 for warm-up/cool-down routines and more details on the beneficial effects of exercise.)

9. Rehearse situations that make you angry, hostile, or anxious so you can learn to respond calmly and with control.

Think about the daily events that get your blood boiling even mildly. An employee is late; the boss asks pointedly if a job is finished when he knows it couldn't be; your office mate in the next cubicle is talking so loud that you can barely concentrate; the kids littered the house with their dirty clothes as if they were Hansel and Gretel leaving a trail of bread crumbs.

Now actually go through the event in your mind as it typically happens; then go through the scene again, this time responding as you'd like to, feeling calm, maybe even laughing at the ridiculous predictability of it all. Next time the event presents itself, try this new way of responding. Don't expect to master it the first time, but eventually you should be able to at least defuse some of that old anger. (See chapter 12 for further discussion of the visualization technique.)

The aim is not to repress anger and other emotions but to stop feeling these negative emotions at the least provocation. A pleasant side-effect of this behavior change is that you liberate a large energy supply for productive use.

10. When under stress, talk encouragingly to yourself; don't undermine your confidence with negative stress-talk.

If a little voice inside you begins to sound like Alice in Wonderland's white rabbit, muttering "Oh dear! Oh dear! I shall be too late!" then it is time to turn to chapter 12 and learn how to talk nicely to yourself. Your internal commentator can either calm you down or stir up anger and anxiety. Even if you are late, you will get any task done more smoothly and comfortably if you approach it confidently instead of feeling as if you're starting out from behind.

11. Practice waiting in line without stress.

This is the hardest lesson for Type A characters. Follow the instructions in chapter 12. Remember a line is not a personal affront to your importance; it is not an example of the world's conspiring to delay your speedy advancement through life. It is nothing more than a wait, a nuisance, perhaps. But you can learn quite useful things to do for yourself and your health while you wait. Try the Ten-Second Stress Fix, do a few exercises, daydream.

12. Enlist help from your family, your friends, in trying to change.

First, this will mean that you are openly committing yourself to trying a few changes, and that commitment makes success more likely.

Second, it is often interactions in the family or in a relationship that make you tense and angry in the first place, or that tend to perpetuate those reactions. So everyone will need to cooperate in modifying shared patterns of response.

However, don't expect others to share your initial enthusiasm about making changes. You're likely to get more cooperation if instead of asking them to *change their ways too* you ask them to help you change some of your attitudes and reactions. To help you, they will soon find themselves responding differently from usual, too. And once family relations improve, once fewer people are flying off the handle, and you stop feeling too pressed for time to enjoy each other's company, then these new satisfactions themselves become the motivation to continue and even make further changes in Type A ways.

13. Find someone you respect who is not Type A to serve as a model.

    Study this person's reactions under stress. See if you can pick up some pointers. Try not to surround yourself with other Type A's who will only reinforce your weakest traits.

14. Master relaxation techniques that you can use on the spot under stress and in longer sessions to unwind.

    No matter how hard you try, there will be times in the day when you will respond with Type A tenseness. So your body will need to repair itself. Relaxation breaks the stress cycle and gives your systems the rest they need to patch you up.

15. Look for the subtle changes that show you are succeeding, and reward yourself.

    Every time you meet your small goal—you get through a day without banging your fist, or you practice muscle relaxation every day for a week—treat yourself to something special. If the treat can be shared with the whole family—a dinner out or a family walk—that's even better. Then the family has a stake in your success and will be more cooperative.

Changing from a Type A to a combination Type A–B does not happen overnight. Don't let yourself feel as time-pressured about changing as you do about living. Revel in the subtle improvements: a new sense of control, confidence, a more cheerful outlook, and an energetic mood. And recognize that if you can get yourself to make a contract about a goal, and carry through on that effort four times in a row, you have passed the biggest hurtle in behavior modification. And you are well on your way to living a longer, happier life.

14
Sleep—
How to Get
the Good Stuff

WE SPEND ONE-THIRD of our lives in a private world of darkness regarded for centuries as a mysterious state beyond our control. It is only in the last couple of decades that sleep researchers have begun to discover that sleep is not a deathlike stupor but a state in which the brain is as active as in waking. And whether we get to sleep and how well we sleep can be influenced by our conscious thoughts and activities while awake.

Getting a good night's sleep is critical to our feeling of well-being. There's nothing like the sensation of stretching in the morning and just knowing that last night's deep sleep has thoroughly refreshed you. You feel as if you can conquer the world, or at least conquer gravity long enough to get up and face the day.

But if you've had a bad night, you feel as stale and lifeless as morning breath. And worse still, you may be jeopardizing your health. A couple of studies have linked insomnia and disturbed sleep to both angina (the chest pain associated with heart disease) and heart attacks. And though no controlled studies have yet been done on chronic sleep troubles and the immune system, we all know that if we haven't slept well we seem more sensitive to aches and pains, less able to fight off colds and viruses, and perhaps to more serious conditions that eventually take hold when immunity weakens. (See chapter 2 for an explanation of the link between cancer and aging to the immune system).

Tiredness can make us more prone to accidents. It can even interfere with our job performance. And it doesn't do great things for relationships if you find yourself fading out just when your lover had hoped you'd perk up.

More than one-third of Americans complain of sleep problems—

and for one out of three of these people, it is, they feel, the most serious problem of their life. Over 20 million prescriptions for sleeping pills are written yearly; over 30 million nonprescription sleeping aids are sold. Most of these potions do little good in aiding insomnia, and for many tired imbibers, this "solution" could really simply be adding to the problem.

There are no rules on exactly how much sleep we need. But there are some rules on how to get what you need to keep feeling healthy, refreshed, and energetic.

Changing Patterns and Improving Sleep Efficiency

No one should lose sleep over not following the "golden rule" of seven to eight hours of sleep a night. It is not a prescription; it is merely an average. Only half the population sleeps seven or eight hours a night. The rest sleep more or less—mostly from five to nine hours—or in several short snoozes.

Sleep needs may be genetically determined. If you've always slept a lot ever since childhood, chances are that there isn't much you can do to change that pattern. However, you should still try experimenting. It is possible that you have not yet hit upon exactly which sleep pattern makes you operate best. And both getting too much sleep as well as getting too little can make you feel sluggish and cranky.

You may be able to get by on less. Napoleon, Thomas Edison, Lyndon Johnson, all were reputed to function dazzlingly on only four hours nightly, though the truth is that they also took naps which brought their total sleep within a twenty-four-hour period closer to the average. Still, people have been able to cut back on their sleep, for a while at least.

Four couples who slept close to the average seven hours managed to cut their sleep by three hours a night for a month. A year later, according to the researcher at the Naval Health Research Center in San Diego, California, who conducted the experiment, they were all sleeping from one-half to two and a half hours less than before the experiment.

The easiest way to try to cut back on your sleeping time is to shave off half an hour of sleep every couple of months. Proceeding gradually gives your body a chance to adjust to the new rhythm. If it doesn't feel right, however, you should stop and try a different length of sleep. Bear in mind that sleep researchers have documented very few cases of people routinely sleeping less than five and a half hours a night.

It could be that what you really need is more sleep, not less. Dr. William Dement, one of the first and foremost of the sleep researchers, told a group of normal sleepers who had no problems with their sleeping habits to sleep one hour more than they usually did. He tested them before and after the new patterns and found all of them to be more alert in the daytime after getting the extra sleep. They had not been operating at peak mental efficiency because they had needed more sleep, but none of them suspected that before the experiment.

There is no shame in sleeping long hours, and there should be no moral judgment attached. Those with Type A, time-pressured leanings may lament the twenty years of our lives that most of us spend in slumber, but some people simply cannot function with less. Albert Einstein didn't apologize for spending nearly half the day in bed, and it didn't hurt his accomplishments either.

Still, for those who wish they had more hours in the day, but can't seem to alter their length of sleep, there is good news. We can improve our sleep efficiency. We can spend less time in bed without sleeping any less by learning methods of falling asleep faster and waking up immediately in the morning. Many of us spend considerably more time in bed than we need to. The tips at the end of this chapter should help you increase sleep efficiency, even if you have no specific sleep complaints.

Personality and Sleeping Time

Short sleepers and long sleepers do not differ in their health, but they do have distinctly different personalities.

Short sleepers (less than six hours) are more efficient, energetic, ambitious people who tend to work hard and keep busy. They are politically conformist, socially adept, practical, and, most important, nonworriers. If they achieve greatness, it is likely as administrators, political leaders, or applied scientists.

Long sleepers (more than nine hours) tend to be nonconformist, critical, anxious, and worried. They are likely to complain about aches and pains. Their greatness tends to manifest itself as "tortured genius," according to research by Dr. Ernest Hartmann, head of the sleep lab at Boston State Hospital.

But the length of time one sleeps does not seem to affect one's success in life. According to two studies, one of over 500 "men of distinction" and another of over 1000 leaders in fields as diverse as art, science, industry, and politics, the successful and famous sleep the same as you and I—an average of eight hours a night, with some sleeping as few as five and some as many as ten.

Early risers seem to have a more positive outlook on life. According to an Australian study of medical students, those who arose an average of forty-five minutes later than the early risers got poorer grades, were more unrealistic about themselves and their capabilities, and complained about their sleep more than the early risers.

Sleep Needs Change with Age

Sleep needs vary not only from person to person but within the same person as he or she ages.

Our sleep patterns tend to get shorter from birth on. Infants sleep sixteen hours a day at first, dreaming about 80 percent of that time. By puberty, teenagers usually are down to nine or ten hours. The decline continues from there.

Nothing else changes so measurably between the ages of twenty and fifty as sleep. We spend 60 percent less time in the deep stages of sleep and we awaken more often in our later years. By age seventy, noises that went unheard in youth readily pierce and disturb the lighter slumber. So the elderly often wind up spending more time in bed but less time asleep. Half of people over sixty experience chronic sleep problems.

Why Do We Sleep?

The one thing sleep researchers can't tell us is why we sleep or what exactly sleep does.

Shakespeare's theory is still the most popular, that sleep "knits up the ravell'd sleave of care." Scientists prefer to call it the recuperative or the restorative theory of sleep. The only trouble is they can't seem to find out what is being restored; there don't seem to be significant changes in the levels of chemicals before and after sleep.

We know that if we don't get sleep, we don't feel right. We get grouchy, depressed, apathetic. Our brains don't seem to function well. We can't solve problems and we lose interest in the world around us. For primitive man, lack of sleep could prove lethal if a predator were nearby. For modern man, sleep troubles can spell danger, too. French studies have shown that sleep-deprived men, when asked to perform a simple task, secrete more epinephrine and norepinephrine than when well-rested. These hormones are linked to increased risks of atherosclerosis and heart attacks (as discussed in greater detail in the heart and stress chapters).

Stages of Sleep—What Each Does

We may not know why we sleep, but we know what the brain goes through when the lights go out.

Sleep follows a rhythmic, cyclic flow of two stages of brain activity: nonrapid eye movement (non-REM) and rapid eye movement (REM) sleep. Non-REM sleep ranges from the lightest, stage 1, to the deepest and, some theorize, the most restful sleep, stage 4.

After about seventy to eighty minutes of the non-REM stages, the REM stage begins. The face and fingertips twitch, snoring ceases since the chin and head muscles lose tone, breathing is irregular, and the eyes dart back and forth beneath the lids. In males, erections occur just before nearly every REM stage from infancy to old age, and last through 95 percent of the REM periods. Women experience increased blood flow to the cervix and the vaginal walls. These phenomena are not affected by whether you've had an orgasm recently nor do they stem from overtly sexual dreams.

Though dreams can occur in all stages of sleep, REM dreams are the most vivid, filled with action and color. The most common colors are green, followed by red, then yellow and blue. The REM stage starts out lasting only ten minutes and gets longer as the night wears on, eventually lasting an hour—nearly as long as a feature film.

Adults complete about five of these ninety-minute cycles a night, adding up to a total of one and a half to two hours of REM sleep. In a lifetime, that means the average person spends five years dreaming. Unfortunately, unless we're awakened in the middle, these spectacular dramas are lost to our waking minds.

Sleep Troubles

Nearly everybody has trouble sleeping at one time or another. About 10 to 20 percent of Americans have prolonged periods of insomnia, with women suffering much more than men.

The problem isn't how much sleep you get. Even insomniacs who think they haven't slept a wink all night have been found when monitored in sleep laboratories to actually get about as much sleep as normal sleepers—sometimes perhaps less than thirty minutes' difference in sleep a night from normal sleepers. The issue with sleep is whether or not it is a pause that refreshes. If it isn't, you've got trouble.

Insomnia

There are two kinds of common sleep dilemmas: when you can't fall asleep in the evening, or when you fall asleep but awaken at 3:00 or 4:00 A.M.—the dark hours of the soul—and can't get back to sleep.

Tensions and worries that accumulate during the day are the primary causes of sleep problems. While getting to the source of your worries is the ultimate solution, there are dozens of simple steps you can take in the meantime to get you the sleep you need to give you the strength to go on. As you'll see at the end of this chapter, there are a host of foods, drinks, drugs, and small habits that may be playing havoc with your sleeping brain waves—while others can be used to ease you into slumber.

Sleep Apnea

Tension, however, is not the only source of sleep problems.

If you feel sleepy during the day—and especially if you smoke heavily, have hypertension, or snore at night—you may suffer from sleep apnea, a condition in which breathing stops for anywhere from a second to as long as a couple of minutes. Once thought to be a rare condition, researchers now figure anywhere from 2 to 5 million Americans are affected by this sleep disorder.

Breathing can come to a halt a few times a night, or as many as 600 times a night. Usually the sufferer has no idea he or she has awakened briefly, but sometimes the apnea actually startles the person awake. In either case, sleep is interrupted and often the result is a feeling of enormous sleepiness the next day.

Serious trouble arises when the patient complains of insomnia and the doctor, unaware of a sleep-apnea condition, prescribes sleeping pills. Sleeping pills depress the respiratory system and can increase the number of apneas that occur at night, making sleep even worse. It may even prove dangerous, depressing breathing reactions so much as to kill a person with severe sleep apnea. Researchers believe the combination may account for certain sudden deaths at night.

Sleep apnea can be cured. In many cases it stems from being over-weight, and losing weight can eliminate the problem. If the windpipe is actually restricted or collapsed, surgery can be performed to open it up. There are also drugs that can stimulate respiration.

In less severe cases, changing sleep positions to your side, not your back, as you would do to eliminate snoring can help prevent obstructing the windpipe. Also learning the relaxation techniques (described in chapter 12, "Learning to Love Stress") can help put you back to sleep quickly.

Snoring

Snorers, you are in illustrious company, from George Washington to Franklin Delano Roosevelt, Winston Churchill to Mussolini. The glamorous and the un- snore. However, if you are also in the company of a very disgruntled and weary bedmate who is kept awake by your nightly throaty serenades, you might try some of the following steps.

- Sleep on your side, not your back—and keep pillows at your back to prevent you from rolling over in your sleep.
- Cut back on smoking and drinking—they irritate mucus membranes and block breathing passageways making snoring worse.
- Use a humidifier or vaporizer—this reduces swollen mucus membranes and reduces the sonorous snore.
- Lose weight—overweight people tend to snore more.
- Check to see if you suffer from allergies—food and hayfever allergies make snoring worse.
- Give your mate earplugs—and make sure he or she gets to bed and to sleep first. Falling asleep next to a snorer is harder than staying asleep.

Tooth Grinding

This grating habit (called "bruxism") can not only drive your bedmate up the wall it can wear down your teeth and damage your gums.

Biofeedback and relaxation exercises during the day to focus muscle relaxation on the jaw can help you relax the jaw at night, too. But if this fails, you might visit a dentist, who should be able to tell instantly if you grind your teeth and who can fit you with a plate to wear at night to bring the grinding to a halt.

Leg Cramps at Night

These cramps can occur at any age, though the elderly and pregnant women seem more prone. While some have thought this wrenching pain that can send you bolt upright clutching frantically at the bulging calf muscle indicates a salt or calcium deficiency, others believe the problem is simply muscular, and can be avoided by stretching before bedtime or changing sleep posture.

Try this calf-muscle stretch to minimize the likelihood of cramping: Stand with your arms outstretched, hands against a wall. Line the toes of one foot up to the wall, keeping the foot flat. Stretch the other foot about three feet behind, also with the foot flat on the floor. Then bending the front leg, keeping the back leg straight, lean gently into the wall, stretching the back calf muscle. Repeat on the other side.

Nightmares and Things That Go Bump . . .

For children, nightmares, night terrors in which they wake up screaming and moaning and terrified, sleepwalking and talking are all not uncommon, and usually are not a sign of any significant emotional disturbance. Most of these sleep disturbances stop by themselves before the child reaches the teen years. Night terrors typically start after age four and end before age eight.

If these sleep disturbances persist into adulthood, however, getting professional advice would be prudent. As many as 4 million Americans may sleepwalk regularly. And it can be dangerous, as the person who sleepwalks may have his eyes open, but usually does not really see. Even for children who will likely outgrow their problems, it is important to take steps to make sure they don't hurt themselves. Don't startle the sleepwalker, but make sure windows and doors in the bedroom are closed to keep him or her from wandering off.

Sleeptalking is a harmless activity that 20 percent of the population engages in and needs no treatment. But if your bedmate's babbles bother your sleep, try gently shifting his position or quietly calling her name and suggesting she stop talking. The suggestion may sink in and you may get the response you want to hear most—blessed silence.

Mythical Sleep Aids

SLEEPING PILLS

Most sleeping pills can put you out in thirty minutes, but only for the first five days. After that they stop working unless you increase the dosage. This merely delays the inevitable, for in five more days the new level won't work. It also makes addiction more likely, and assures there will be an unpleasant, drowsy hangover effect during the day that can make getting to sleep the next night even more difficult.

Furthermore, though sleeping pills can get you to sleep, most cannot keep you asleep. Hypnotics distort the natural stages of sleep, repressing REM and deep stage 4 sleep. When you stop taking the pills, you can experience rebound insomnia and also rebound REM sleep—intense, often frightening, dreams.

Even over-the-counter sleeping aids have not been pronounced either safe or effective by the Food and Drug Administration.

Sleeping pills may have use in special traumatic circumstances for very short periods. But in most cases of insomnia, they will only cause more discomfort than they can ease.

ALCOHOL

For many, a little nightcap seems to help them relax and fall asleep fast. But if you find you are awakening in the night, or rising in the morning still not feeling refreshed, it may be your solution that is the problem.

Alcohol interferes with REM and stage 4 sleep and so may cause you to wake up in the night or simply not get as much of the restful sleep you need. Its excellent diuretic properties may also awaken you in the night to hurry off to the bathroom.

In addition, spirits aggravate sleep apnea and can even induce it in those who usually have no more sleep problems than snoring. Alcohol can lengthen those usually short periods when you stop breathing, which disrupts your sleep. In more serious cases, the oxygen deprivation can lead to memory loss, personality changes, cardiac arrhythmias (irregular heartbeats), and even heart failure.

FOODS THAT LET YOU DOWN AND KEEP YOU UP

You know that coffee, tea, and colas can keep you up. But you may not realize that there is caffeine in a number of other sources: chocolate, many cold capsules, aspirin compounds, and over-the-counter pain relievers, including Anacin, Bromo-Seltzer, Empirin, Midol, Excedrin among others.

Furthermore, it isn't just that swallow of caffeine right before bed that stirs you up, but the quantities you consume all day. Caffeine's stimulating effects build up and linger in the body from seven to twenty-four hours.

Dieter's Dilemma

Finally, you've stuck to a strict diet, you feel proud of yourself, but still you find yourself staring wide-eyed at the ceiling above the bed. Why?

It would seem that it is almost as difficult to fall asleep on an empty stomach as it is on a full one. Dieters should save enough calories in their daily allotment for a light bedtime snack. It can help you feel calm and drowsy.

Nature's Sleeping Potions

Good sex is an excellent soporific. Reaching orgasm seems to ease one into sleep whether you want to rest or not.

If you're not in the mood, you might try nature's other sleeping pill, L-tryptophan. It is an amino acid that occurs naturally in milk products and tuna fish, and is one of the building blocks of serotonin, the brain chemical associated with sleep. Skim milk is your best best, as it is lower in fat than regular milk, easier to digest, and therefore less likely to cause any digestive upsets in the night. (Milk also contains calcium and magnesium, two minerals that seem to soothe the nervous system.) Hot chocolate, however, may prove a wash as the caffeine in the chocolate could cancel the soothing effects of the milk.

L-tryptophan is also available in tablets. Sleep researchers say that one gram taken a little more than half an hour before bedtime can help make you drowsy. However, here, as with most vitamins and minerals, you are safest going after the chemical as it occurs naturally in food.

Naps

Salvador Dali, the Spanish artist and flamboyant eccentric, used to claim that he would sit in a chair, put a tin plate on the floor at his feet, and hold a spoon over the plate. As he fell asleep, the spoon would slip from his fingers, hit the plate with a clatter, and awaken him. No matter, Dali insisted, for he claimed to be totally refreshed by the sleep he got in just those seconds between the spoon's leaving his fingers and its hitting the plate.

Researchers used to believe that any nap less than two hours and running through an entire non-REM and REM sleep cycle would not be restful. This is no longer accepted as true.

Most of the well-known short sleepers manage their four-hour nights by taking daytime naps. Winston Churchill swore by his regular twenty-minute catnaps. A study of women who felt nervous and fatigued during the day found that about two-thirds of them felt much better after incorporating short naps into their days.

However, naps are not considered a good idea if you have trouble sleeping at night. Most people seem to prefer to sleep one-third of the twenty-four-hour period in one unbroken sleep session. If the only way you can catch sleep is in a nap, fine. But if you want to get back on a normal, nightly schedule, leave the naps for cats.

Sleep Learning

If you've got a little tape recording blaring "Bonjour. Comment-allez vous?" under your pillow at night, turn it off and let yourself sleep in peace.

Although people were spending an estimated $10 million a year on tapes and records at the peak of the sleep-learning craze in the 1950s, trying to learn everything from French to salesmanship and weight-loss willpower in their sleep, studies since show no evidence that any of it works.

The only learning that takes place during sleep is negative learning, learning not to become alarmed by innocuous noises. The brain continuously registers environmental stimuli as we sleep, but we learn which to filter out and which are significant enough to merit waking up. This screening ability is called "the baby's cry" phenomenon because parents can sleep through the thunder of a two-ton garbage truck right outside their window yet awaken when they hear the whimper of their tiny baby way down the hall.

Get the Most Out of Your Sleep: Increase Your Sleep Efficiency

Even if you have no trouble sleeping, the following advice can help you increase your sleep efficiency, get you the most refreshing rest from the fewest hours in bed.

And if you, like most of us, have difficulty from time to time falling asleep or feeling your most energetic the next day, these tips on habits, postures, and approaches to sleep can help you, as they've helped others, get a good night's sleep.

How to Get to Sleep

1. Don't wait for the night to relax.

    Take a few minutes out several times during the day to close your eyes, breathe deeply, and relax. (See chapter 12, "Learning to Love Stress," for the Ten-Second Stress Fix and other relaxation techniques.) Otherwise tension may build to such intense levels that it can take all night to unwind.

2. Exercise in the late afternoon or early evening.

    Athletes have been shown to have more of the deepest and perhaps most relaxing stage sleep than nonathletes. But timing is crucial. To deepen and lengthen your sleep, you should work out in the late afternoon or early evening. Morning exercise may relax your afternoon, but its calming effects will likely be gone by bedtime; and exercising too late in the evening will be stimulating rather than calming.

3. Good sex can mean good sleep.

    The above caution about exercising at bedtime does not apply to sex. Even if lovemaking is physically active, if it is also pleasurable and satisfying, it is an excellent soporific.

    Even if you are alone, this remains an option. The same sleep-inducing chemicals are released no matter how you reach orgasm.

4. Avoid caffeine—the obvious and not-so-obvious sources.

    The effects of caffeine build up throughout the day and linger into the night. So cut out this stimulant beginning at least seven hours before bedtime. You'll find caffeine in coffee, teas, colas, chocolate, many cold capsules, and aspirin compounds and over-the-counter pain relievers.

5. Dieters need a nibble.

Dieters often have trouble getting to sleep. Those who are gaining weight sleep better than those trying to lose. So save a few calories for a bedtime snack.

6. Sip warm milk or chomp on a very small tuna and lettuce sandwich.

Milk, lettuce, and tuna fish all contain L-tryptophan, an amino acid that is a natural sleeping aid. They also contain calcium and magnesium, two minerals which seem to calm the nervous system.

7. A nightcap may help . . . then again . . .

A bit of rum in warm milk or a glass of sherry may relax you enough to help you sleep. But don't have a nightcap if you've already had a few drinks earlier. Too much alcohol can disrupt your sleep and dreams (see discussion on alcohol's effects below).

8. Go to sleep at the same hour each night.

Keeping your bedtime and hour of awakening as regular as possible—give or take an hour—prepares you for sleep. Wild and crazy weekends, with late nights and lazy mornings can upset your weekday schedule, too. Even if one night you get to bed later than usual, you should try waking up at the normal time anyway so you won't have trouble the following night. You may have a slightly sleepy day, but that's usually better than several sleepness nights.

9. Don't nap.

Sure, you're tired because you couldn't fall asleep last night. But if you nap, you won't be able to get to sleep tonight, and the cycle will continue. Resist the daytime shut-eye and get back on a regular schedule.

This admonition does not apply if you are not having trouble getting to sleep at night. If a nap refreshes you without keeping you from sleeping at the normal time, doze on.

10. Start winding down well before bedtime.

Take a warm bath, listen to soothing music, spend at least fifteen minutes doing something that completely relaxes your mind and body.

Practice visualizing peaceful images—gorgeous deserted beaches with lapping waves and pure white sand, a pond, stream, gently sloping green hillside beneath fluffy white clouds floating in an azure sky. Don't worry about being original; seek the soothing.

11. Try eye rolls and muscle relaxation.

As you lie in bed with eyes closed, roll your eyes upward. People in deep sleep turn their eyes upward. It is the sleep position for the eyes. Assuming this position may help trigger the brain that it is time for sleep.

Then try muscle relaxation, tensing and releasing every muscle from forehead to toe, and thinking about all the tightness and anxiety flowing out of every pore of your body, out and away. (Again these techniques are laid out in chapter 12.)

12. Keep out of bed unless you're ready to sleep.

Insomniacs spend too much time in bed, doing things other than sleeping. It builds up in your mind an association of the bed with activity and wakefulness rather than rest. If you have trouble sleeping, don't watch TV, read, or make phone calls from bed. Treat it as a quiet haven for sleep only.

13. Get up if you can't fall asleep.

If you can't fall asleep within about fifteen minutes, get up and do something relaxing but constructive until you feel sleepy. The worst thing you can do for yourself is to lie there and fret about another sleepless night.

If you're too worried about a problem even to read a novel, then sit down and fill out this form:

What's Bothering Me	Action Plan for Tomorrow
1.	1.
2.	2

Don't write a novel, just get to the heart of it, say what's eating at you enough to keep you awake. And then decide to take one small, specific step tomorrow (two at the most) to get a handle on the problem—a small first step, not the ultimate solution. It helps put problems in perspective and puts you back in control. You will feel as if you have accomplished something simply by laying out this plan of action. And perhaps now you can pick up that novel and allow yourself to relax into sleep.

How to Stay Asleep

1. Keep the room cool.

The best sleeping temperatures seem to be about 60 to 65 degrees F. If the room is too cold, under 55 degrees F, for some reason, dreams tend to be highly emotional and unpleasant. If the room is too hot, you'll wake up more frequently.

2. Don't take that puff.

Nicotine craving can actually awaken you from a deep sleep with the desire to smoke a cigarette. Heavy smokers take longer to fall asleep and have less REM and stage 4 sleep than nonsmokers.

However, within three days of quitting smoking, a former smoker will find sleep improved. And within two weeks, sleep returns to normal, restful patterns.

3. Avoid alcohol for a few days.

Though a nightcap may seem to put you to sleep faster, it may disrupt sleep later on. Alcohol suppresses REM and stage 4 sleep. And it doesn't take getting drunk to do the mischief—even one or two drinks can create later sleep troubles. So if you find yourself waking up in the night, you might try cutting out the booze or at least stopping with a couple of glasses of wine at dinner.

4. Steer clear of caffeine.

Even if it doesn't keep you from falling asleep, caffeine can make you wake up later on. Like other stimulants, it seems to reduce stage 4 sleep.

5. Keep noises down.

We never fully get used to loud noises in the night. Our brain registers them even if we don't awaken and that disturbs our sleep. So if you live on a noisy street, try to shut out the racket by closing windows or setting up your own gentle but constant background noise—the whirring of a fan, or a continuous-playing cassette of ocean waves or white noise.

6. Have a soothing phrase ready to whisper to yourself.

Rehearse in advance how you will calmly get back to sleep if you should awaken in the night.

As you look at the clock and see it is still the dark hour of the soul, say something soothing to yourself. Not: "Oh, Lord, I'll never get back to sleep." Rather: "Ah, still some time to sleep; I'll just take a few deep breaths, feel myself getting calmer, my mind going blank, and I'll relax back into sleep." As you say it, breathe deeply, and let go.

How to Wake Up Refreshed

1. Your sleep postures affect daytime moods.

If you've slept badly or peculiarly, you wake up feeling achy and out of sorts. Though you shift positions many times throughout the night, you can guide yourself to postures that will make you feel best in the morning.

If you awaken with backaches, it may be because you're sleeping on your stomach, which curves the spine. It's better to lie on your back, putting a pillow under the feet or knees to further ease the pressure on the spine. Lying on either side with a pillow between the knees can also take pressure off the back.

2. Pick a pillow that molds as you move.

Big thick foam pillows can give you a stiff neck. You want a pillow that keeps your head and neck on a straight horizontal line with your spine. Down pillows work best. They can be bunched up for more thickness when you lic on your side. The pillow should fill a space as wide as the span from your shoulder to your neck to keep the spine aligned. And they can be pushed flat as you lie on your back or stomach when you actually need no pillow at all.

3. Mattress mystique—pick something firm that also gives.

Nighttime is not the right time to do penance and sleep on boards. Your mattress, while being firm, should also allow your body to follow its natural contours so the muscles can relax. A firm mattress prevents body parts from sagging and allows you to keep your posture straight without straining. Test them out by lying down before you buy. Sarah Bernhardt slept in her coffin. You have to find what suits you.

4. Shun sleeping pills.

Though they can put you to sleep within thirty minutes, most sleeping pills distort the natural stages of sleep (interfering with REM and stage 4 cycles) and lose effectiveness after about five days. They can also leave you with a groggy daytime hangover.

5. Wake up with a headache? Quit playing ostrich with the covers.

If you wake up in the morning, groan at the early light, and pull the covers back over your head for an extra snooze, you're asking for trouble. Carbon dioxide will build up under there, depriving the brain of oxygen and resulting in a headache.

6. Choose light meals and a brisk walk to spark energy after a sleepless night.

If you didn't sleep well last night, make sure you eat light but healthy foods and use the quick-stress-fix routine often throughout the day to minimize the strain on your digestive and nervous systems. If you need energy, drink extra water and take a brisk walk—don't rely on caffeine.

7. Remind yourself that lack of sleep won't kill you.

No matter how bad you may feel, bear in mind that no one ever died from lack of sleep. Insomniacs may have killed others, perhaps, but that is a matter for some other book. You will not only live, but if you follow these tips, tonight will be better.

These tips for getting the most out of your sleeping hours have worked for others and they can work for you. It may take a few days to settle into some of the new habits and patterns, so be patient. You hear? Hey, wake up. Are you paying attention? Good.

Now, sweet dreams.

15
Diet for Health— Eat Better, Live Longer

EATING RIGHT DOESN'T just make you feel better, it could add as much as eleven years to your life according to some federal nutrition experts.

Poor diets—which include eating the "wrong foods" as well as too much of the "right foods"—play a part in the evolution of nearly every disease you can name.

- Too much fat and cholesterol in the diet can lead to clogged coronary arteries, heart attacks, and strokes.
- Too much fat and too little fruits and vegetables have been implicated in breast, stomach, esophogeal, and colon cancers.
- And simply eating too much of both the "wrong" and "right" foods, which makes us fat, can trigger and aggravate everything from arthritis and diabetes to hypertension, heart disease, and cancer.

But just as poor eating habits can jeopardize our health, good habits can improve it.

The General Good-Health Diet

Most Americans have a diet that breaks down as 46 percent carbohydrates, 42 percent fat, and 12 percent protein. According to the National Academy of Sciences, the breakdown should be closer to 60 percent carbohydrates, 30 percent fat, and 10 percent protein. The most critical changes most of us need to make fall into four categories:

losing weight, cutting fats and cholesterol, cutting back on salt, and increasing fiber as well as decreasing refined sugars.

And the diet plans that follow explain exactly how to make those four basic changes, without making mealtime a bore.

There are also some diet tips for combating colds, preventing brittle bones, and preparing for sports events.

What to Do	Helps Prevent
Lose weight	Heart disease
	Diabetes
	Arthritis
	Cancer
Cut fats, cholesterol	Heart disease
	Cancer
Cut back on salt	Hypertension
	Heart disease
	Certain cancers
Increase fiber, decrease refined sugars	Diabetes
	Heart disease
	Cancer

The Great Weighting Game—How to Win at Losing

There are about 7 million severely obese people in the United States, 13 million moderately obese, and 80 million just overweight (which covers all who tip the scales at more than 20 percent above their ideal weight—see later in this chapter for how to figure out yours).

We do not all bear the extra poundage equally. Women are more likely than men to be overweight. Poor men are less likely than middle-class men to be overweight, while poor women are more likely to be heavy than their wealthier counterparts.

Many of us have tried, will keep on trying, anything and everything to shed that extra burden we carry around. But the drugs and fad diets just don't work, and worse, they can be dangerous.

That does not mean you can't lose weight. And it isn't simply a matter of willpower. There are approaches and techniques you can learn that help you lose more with less difficulty.

First, you have to understand how fat builds up and what really works at breaking it down. Armed with that understanding of the mechanisms behind weight loss, you have a much greater chance of taking it off and keeping it off for good.

Why Lose Weight?

As you know from chapter 6, "Heart Disease," the body needs three-quarters of a mile of blood vessels for every pound of fat—with 20 pounds of extra fat, the heart has to work overtime pumping blood through 15 extra miles of pipes every 13 seconds, 4000 extra miles an hour. So it is not surprising that being overweight makes one more susceptible to everything from heart disease and cancer to arthritis and diabetes. In addition to that direct physical strain there is the psychological burden—for many, the extra weight is a constant embarrassment, causing constant stress. And, as you know too, that can increase the odds on contracting nearly all illnesses.

If you get close to the average weight for your size, chances are you will live longer. Even those already ill, with such diseases as breast cancer, have been shown to live longer if they keep their weight down. In mice studies it has been shown that those fed half the calories live twice as long.

But diets must be sensible if we are to stay healthy. And the first things to digest are the facts.

Why We Get Fat—the Theories

Here is one certainty: if you eat more than your body burns up, you gain weight. But why can some people load their plates without overloading their systems, while others seem to put on weight just by looking at food? The experts still are not quite sure, but here are some possible explanations:

Fat Cells

You can't get fat without fat cells. Unfortunately, we all have them, around 25 billion of them. The number of fat cells in the body can increase, but it will never decrease. This means that if, as a baby or at any other time in your life you become quite fat, you will produce more fat cells. And even if you later lose weight, you won't reduce the number of fat cells, only the content of each fat cell.

The fat content of a given cell depends upon how many calories are made available for storage as fat; that is, how many more calories you eat than you burn. And each cell itself can swell up to three times its normal size. This makes it very easy to regain weight you have lost, and it may help explain why so many earnest dieters bounce up and down in weight.

Set Point

Another theory about weight control is that we all have a "set point," a thermostat in the brain that controls appetite, telling us when to eat and when to stop. According to this theory, the set point is determined at birth and firmed up in youth, but it may also be consciously altered in adulthood.

You can fool your set point into registering "full" even when you eat less than normal. For example, if you eat very slowly, the signal that you are full (which usually takes about twenty minutes from the time you begin eating to register) goes off in the brain before you've eaten as much as usual. High-fiber, low-calorie foods such as carrots and celery, other vegetables and fruits as well as grains keep you chewing longer than sweet or high-fat foods and, of course, yield good nutrients.

Exercise—for the "Even When I Eat Less, I Can't Lose" Folks

If you have a friend who says that after the first couple of weeks of a diet she just can't lose any weight no matter how little she eats, what is your first reaction? You suspect she's cheating, right?

Not necessarily. Food may not be the problem, exercise could be— or rather the lack of it.

Cutting back on food is sometimes not enough. The body has evolved means to protect us from starvation. When you cut back drastically on your calories, an alarm goes off in the body cells. They react as if these tiny meals may be their last, and they slow down their basal metabolic rate—the rate cells use up calories when you're at rest—to conserve energy. Your metabolism can slow down by nearly one-half. So even if you're eating much less, your cells are not burning it all up.

And if you get exasperated and go off the diet altogether while your cells are still slowed down, you may find yourself gaining even faster than you would ordinarily.

How do you get around this?

Exercise. Vigorous movement does more than simply burn up calories. It speeds up your metabolism not just while you're exercising but for as long as twenty-four hours afterward as well.

Weight loss from exercise alone is slow, but it is more likely to be permanent than simply dieting. And when exercise and low-calorie diets are combined, the effects are much more rapid and satisfying than either tactic alone. As you lose the fat in cells beneath the skin, exercise helps tighten you up in a shapely way instead of allowing the skin to go loose and flabby. People who exercise and diet lose more body fat and less lean muscle tissue than those who simply diet. And the tightening up from exercise makes the results of a diet visible much more quickly and dramatically.

Exercise brings other benefits for those trying to lose weight:

- A workout tends to depress, not increase, your appetite.
- And it does anything but depress your mood. It stimulates the release of hormones that are the body's natural mood elevators. So you begin to feel better about yourself, more confident about sticking to your goals, and less likely to feel the impulse to drown your sorrows in food.
- Once you develop more muscle cells, your body will burn more calories than it used to just to keep going. Even at rest, muscle cells are thought to be more active than fat cells.

Exercise can make you look trimmer even if you don't actually lose weight. You are losing fat cells and gaining muscle cells. Muscle does weigh more than fat, but since muscle is also more compact than fat, you may find your belt going in a couple of notches and your dress size moving down several numbers on the rack, regardless of what the scale reads.

Besides, exercise feels lousy on a full stomach. You can't run or dance within several hours of a big meal—so committing yourself to an exercise regimen will also add to your incentive to stick to small, easy-to-digest meals. You might even plan the timing of your exercise to make the most of this. Early evening exercise means you have to have a small lunch, and it dampens your appetite (and speeds up your metabolism) for dinner.

How to Figure Your "Ideal" Weight

If you are confused by the changing height/weight charts issued by the insurance companies and if you can't figure out what they mean by

"Height with two-inch heels" (Does that make you two inches taller than you really are? one inch? Both are possible.) or "Weight with street clothes" (Does that mean summer or winter clothes? Allow for two pounds, one pound, half a pound? All are possible.), here's a simple method to find the healthiest weight for your height.

For men. Take your height in inches and multiply by 4. Then subtract 127. For example, if you are 5 feet 11 inches then you figure as follows: height of 71 inches × 4 = 284 − 127 = 157.

For women. Take your height in inches and multiply by 3.5. Then subtract 107. For example, if you are 5 feet 5 inches than you figure as follows: height of 65 inches × 3.5 = 227.5 − 107 = 120.5.

If you are large-boned or very muscular, your ideal weight may be a few pounds more than this equation allows.

No Lumps, No Grumps—15 Tips for Diet Success

Behind every theory about why we gain weight there is still only one bedrock truth about how to lose—you must consume fewer calories than you burn. To be exact, you must eat fewer than ten calories a day per pound of body weight in order to lose pounds.

Here's how you can go about eating less without feeling irritable and deprived.

1. Cut back on calories gradually rather than dramatically slashing your intake right at first.

   If you proceed gradually then you are less likely to set off the "starvation alarm" in your cells that makes them burn food more slowly and makes losing that much more painstaking. It also helps you to change your eating habits permanently so your weight won't be bouncing up and down. Try cutting out desserts the first week. Then alcohol, the second. By the third week you can start making your food portions a bit smaller. And by the fourth week you can change the kinds of foods you eat to lower-fat, lower-calorie selections.

2. After you set small goals each week (as explained above) and reach them, celebrate.

   But don't celebrate with food. Treat yourself to a movie or a massage—something sensual and pleasant that does not involve eating.

3. Try three small meals (with controlled snacks in between, if necessary) instead of fewer big meals; and drink plenty of water.

Studies show that eating three small meals spread throughout the day makes it easier to lose weight than eating the same number of calories jammed into only one or two meals. Overweight people tend to eat fewer meals than thin people; they often skip breakfast, pick at lunch, and then have a whopping dinner.

Part of the explanation may be that eating actually increases your metabolic rate temporarily. That accounts for the warm sensation you experience after a meal. Thus, eating several small meals may actually burn off more calories than one large meal.

In addition, spreading meals throughout the day means that you don't let yourself get absolutely famished and so desperate that you'll allow yourself to eat anything, such as a handy candy bar.

Keep a glass of water close by throughout the day. It not only helps fill your stomach and keeps you from reaching for more caloric things, but it seems to give you energy as well.

4. Keep off the scales after the first week.

The first week of a diet is encouraging since the pounds usually drop quickly. But as this loss is mostly water, the dramatic weight loss stops after the second or third week. This is the point when many get discouraged and quit. Don't use the scales as the only measure. Check your body—pinch yourself gently to see if the folds of fat are getting thinner; that's what really counts. People don't look at you and see numbers on a bathroom scale; they look and either they see fat or they don't.

5. Start a regular exercise regimen.

You've read the reasons above. Now turn to chapters 10 and 11 for advice on how to get moving.

6. Don't wear tight clothes.

First of all, they're an irritating reminder that you aren't exaclty where you'd like to be in the weight department. And who needs reminders?

But, more important, tight clothing inhibits movement and you want to do everything you can to encourage yourself to move— movement means calories are burning and flesh is trimming up.

7. Try on old clothes that used to be tight to see how you're doing, but as with the scales, you shouldn't do it every day—maybe once a week.

The body changes slowly, especially the thighs and waistline. So be patient. But noticing that clothes are beginning to fit better can be a powerful spur to continue the battle of the bulge.

8. Tell others you are on a diet—commit yourself publicly.

You don't have to tell everyone you meet, but if you tell your friends and housemates that you are on a diet, it makes it harder to stray.

Ask for their help to stay on the diet. And don't get angry with them if they live up to the bargain and try to save you from that chocolate chip cookie that looks like it has your name on it.

9. Before you go out to eat, rehearse in your mind what may happen to tempt you off your diet and rehearse how you will resist.

Imagine yourself in the restaurant, looking at the menu or hearing the waiter announce the dishes. Tell yourself how tempting the simple chicken and fish dishes will sound and how unappealing the rich, cream-laden dishes will seem. Hear yourself actually ordering the fish. Reach for the water glass, not the bread basket. And practice saying, "I'm so full I couldn't even think about dessert."

10. Recognize that you will go off the diet at some point—it is inevitable—but that does not mean you have failed, nor does it mean you should just forget the whole thing.

All right, so you couldn't resist that cookie calling out to be eaten, and maybe the cookie had a brother or sister and you couldn't bear the idea of breaking up the family. But just because you've slipped up this once doesn't mean all is lost.

Your body does not recognize a diet as an all-or-nothing proposition. It only knows what goes in. If the will is weak today, don't waste time feeling guilty. Just wake up tomorrow with even stronger resolve to stick to the plan. Maybe you've lost a day—big deal. You didn't gain all this extra weight in a day and you can't lose it that quickly either. Any behavior change, especially one as fundamental as eating habits, has its ups and downs.

11. Never eat standing up, out of a bag or a box, or while watching TV. Set out even the simplest meal on a plate and sit down to relish it.

If you eat while doing something else, you aren't keeping track of how much you're eating and you aren't concentrating on the flavors either. So afterward, you might still feel hungry even if you've had enough.

Savor all meals, eat slowly, and make them look attractive. Cut vegetables at appealing angles, lay them out decoratively on the plate. You shouldn't feel as if you're denying yourself just because you're on a diet. You can treat yourself well without gorging.

12. If you feel an urge for something sweet, take a bite of something sour or go brush your teeth.

A taste of lemon or pickle often curbs the desire for something sweet, and neither lemons nor pickles have any calories to speak of. Failing that, toothpaste can make your mouth feel fresh, and besides nothing tastes good after you've just brushed your teeth.

13. Avoid temptations: do not buy forbidden foods, even "for guests or the rest of the family"; keep out of the kitchen as much as possible; and turn off the TV if you want to help turn off your appetite.

Even if the kitchen is stocked only with the bare healthy essentials, it is best to stay away from temptation and the reminder of food.

As for the television, you'll have to decide for yourself whether you're strong enough to resist the ads, one-fourth of which during prime time and weekend-daytime are for food—nearly half of those are for sweet, basically nonnutritious foods. Why torture yourself?

14. If the craving for something sweet becomes overwhelming, take one bite of a sweet treat and relish it. Throw the rest away quickly so you won't be tempted further.

One bite can satisfy that powerful lusting for the forbidden that occasionally hits without throwing your diet out of whack. You don't need to eat the whole thing.

15. Forget about drugs and fad diets. They don't work as well as a modified, healthy, all-around diet, and they can do you considerable harm.

Drugs and diet pills just don't work in the long run. Studies (such as the one of 120 obese women conducted by researchers at Pennsylvania State University) show that people who rely solely on changing their behavior—rather than on appetite-suppressant drugs or even a combination of the drugs and behavior changes—are the only ones who will have kept the weight off one year later.

Furthermore, diet drugs are dangerous. Diet aids containing the stimulant phenylpropanolamine HCL have been reported in medical journals to damage the heart.

And fad diets don't work for long either. No one can spend a lifetime on cottage cheese, or fructose, or heaven knows what else. Liquid protein or powdered-protein diets can be a great strain on the heart, not to mention the immune system, as they cannot supply all the vitamins and minerals and bulk the body needs to stay healthy. Seventeen people are known to have died so far on these drastic diets. No point being skinny if you make yourself sick, or worse.

A modest but well-rounded diet is the best bet for healthy slimming. However, "well-rounded" in light of what nutritionists now know may not be what you grew up thinking it was.

Diet to Lower Fat and Cholesterol

To lower your blood levels of cholesterol, it is more important to lower your intake of fatty foods than foods high in cholesterol. However, if you are at high risk, you will want to do both.

And while it may be slightly more important to reduce saturated fats (animal fats that are solid at room temperature) than polyunsaturated fats (vegetable fats that are liquid at room temperature), for the best health results you will need to lower both.

HOW TO CUT FAT

1. Eat less red meat, which is high in fat, and more poultry and fish, which are excellent, lower-calorie sources of protein.

    If you are being very strict, bear in mind that the lighter the fish or the poultry, the less fat it contains. Dark red salmon, for example, is one of the richest fishes. Ducks and geese are the fattiest of poultry.
2. Make at least one meal a week with neither meat nor fish but rather vegetable protein.

    You need to combine two different vegetables in order to get a complete protein (as meat or fish provides). That is the reason such dishes as black beans and rice, or peanut butter and whole-grain bread, or cheese and noodles seem to go naturally together. They provide a much cheaper and lower-fat source of protein than red meat.
3. Don't fry foods when baking, broiling, or stewing will do.

    If you must use some fat in cooking, try sesame and other light vegetable oils (even for basting), instead of butter, lard, palm and coconut oil, which are the most highly saturated of the oils. (Note: Coconut and palm oil are used in powdered coffee lighteners.)
4. Use lemon juice or a dash of tarragon vinegar or other herbs on vegetables instead of butter to add moisture and flavor. Wine in cooking will do the same for main courses; heating burns off the alcohol and the calories of the wine. Garlic and onions will also supply richness of flavor and moisture without calories.
5. Cut back on but do not shy away from milk and cheese products completely.

Children especially should not forgo milk. While milk and cheese and other milk products may be high in fat and calories, there are skim-milk versions of most products that are just as high in nutrients with less fat. Even for adults—especially those growing older and in need of calcium for their increasingly brittle bones— skim milk should be part of the diet.

6. Eat yogurt; you can even use it as a substitute for sour cream.

In addition to being a low-fat protein and vitamin source, yogurt may have something in it which acts to lower cholesterol levels in the blood.

HOW TO CUT CHOLESTEROL

1. First you have to know where to find it. Cholesterol is in foods of animal origin—milk, cheese, eggs, poultry. The highest sources are eggs and organ meats. Aim to keep daily intake below 500 milligrams of cholesterol.

2. Eggs are very high in cholesterol, though they have probably gotten a nastier reputation than they deserve. Unless you are at high risk, you don't have to avoid them completely, as they are a cheap, low-calorie protein source; but adults probably shouldn't have more than three a week—fewer if you already have high cholesterol— and children, seven.

   To cut back, try eating more white than yolk (give your pet one of the yolks of every two eggs you crack). The white of an egg has more protein and fewer than one-third the calories of the yolk: 17 calories and 3.6 grams of protein versus the yolk's 59 calories and 2.7 grams of protein. Better still, the white contains no fats or cholesterol, while the yolk contains 252 milligrams of cholesterol and much fat.

3. Organ meats, such as liver, brain, heart, kidney, are very high in cholesterol: brain has 572 milligrams of cholesterol per ounce, heart has 70 to 80; kidney, 107; liver, 125–213; sweetbreads, 133.

4. Shellfish have the highest cholesterol levels of any of the fish, but they are still much lower in cholesterol than equivalent portions of red meat and they are much lower in fat and calories.

   A dozen oysters or two small lobsters contain about as much cholesterol as one egg. Three ounces of crab meat—about the size of a medium crab cake—contains under 100 calories.

5. The white meat of chicken has no cholesterol and less fat than dark meat, which itself has very little of either.

6. Nuts are high in fat (more unsaturated than saturated), but they have no cholesterol.

7. Americans now devote about 42 percent of their diet to fat; the National Academy of Sciences recmends that it should be lowered to 30 percent. And Nathan Pritikin, originator of the abstemious diet that bears his name, says that by lowering the diet to only 10 percent, you can reduce cholesterol levels in the blood 27 percent in three to four weeks.

Cut the Salt Habit—a Whole Lot of Shaking Going On

A couple of decades ago several cross-cultural studies turned up the information that tribes with very little salt in their diets, such as the Solomon Islanders, have very little hypertension, while industrialized societies such as Japan, where salt-preserved fish and sodium-rich soy sauce are especially popular, suffer epidemics of the disorder.

The theory is that salt can trigger hypertension—maybe not in everyone but at least in those who are genetically more sensitive to salt than others. The only problem is that no one knows in advance who is sensitive or how much salt may trigger the disorder. That means that the safest bet is for everyone to cut back on salt.

For most of us there is no danger in cutting back on salt. We eat about twenty times more than we need to maintain the proper fluid balance in all our bodily cells. A hamburger with mustard and a pickle, French fries with ketchup, and a milk shake contain nearly 4 grams of salt, practically the recommended intake for a whole day in one meal. The salt found naturally in foods amounts to all we need.

And while some still question whether salt can trigger hypertension, no one disputes that salt will dangerously aggravate the conditions of those who already suffer from the disorder. For those with hypertension, the aim is not only to reduce salt (sodium) intake but also to increase the potassium consumed. It is the balance of these two minerals that helps prevent or lower high blood pressure.

Foods high in potassium include fresh fruits, especially citrus fruits and bananas, vegetables, especially tomatoes, milk, beans, and meats.

HOW TO CUT SALT

1. Avoid or reduce consumption of foods that are high in salt: smoked or luncheon meats such as bacon, corned beef, bologna, ham, hot dogs, sausage, salt pork.

    Smoked fish such as lox, smoked oysters.

    Condiments such as soy sauce, ketchup, mustard, bouillon cubes.

Cheeses, with Roquefort, Camembert, cheese spreads, and most processed cheeses being the saltiest.

Briny foods such as pickles, sauerkraut, olives.

Canned soups and frozen dinners.

Read food ingredient labels. Be on the lookout for any of the following names for salt: sodium chloride, sodium bicarbonate, sodium nitrate, monosodium glutamate, sodium propionate.

2. Don't add salt while cooking.

Salt can leach the vitamins and minerals out of foods into the cooking liquid, so you are not only gaining unnecessary salt but also losing important nutrients.

3. Don't bring the salt shaker to the table.

If you actually have to get up from your meal to go to the kitchen and get the salt shaker, you may think twice before adding it.

4. Buy salt shakers with tiny holes.

An Australian study by researchers at the University of New South Wales, showed that more than three-quarters of people who add salt at the table never even taste their food first. And all people used less salt when the shaker had smaller holes. (The hole size should be no less than three square millimeters, or people seem tempted to remove the lid or enlarge the holes and use even more.)

5. Use lemon and spices on foods you would normally salt.

Herbs such as parsley, tarragon, rosemary, oregano, thyme, dill, basil, and so on enhance flavor, as salt does, without the ill effects. Lemon, pepper, and paprika seem to bring out the natural saltiness in foods.

Increase Fiber and Carbohydrates, Decrease Sugar

Most of us grew up believing that carbohydrates or starches would make us fat. But it turns out that for all of us—and especially for those who want to lose weight—the best bet is to eat more of them not less. Complex carbohydrates have important nutrients themselves, and increasing their share in our diet can help us decrease the real culprits: fats and sugars.

1. Avoid processed foods and soft drinks.

These two changes in Americans' diets since the turn of the century are primarily responsible for our consuming less starch and more sugar than we used to. (At the turn of the century Americans' diets contained 68 percent carbohydrates and 32 percent sugars; today starches are down to 47 percent and sugars are up to 53 percent.)

2. Munch carrots and celery throughout the day whenever you feel like having a snack.

   These high-fiber foods have almost no calories and they keep your mouth and stomach occupied. For weight watchers, these are free foods—you can eat as much as you want.

3. Choose whole-grain breads, pastas, and flours whenever you can.

   In the last decade there has been a dazzling increase in the choices of fiber-rich whole-grain foods—breads, cereals, and even pastas. Each small selection helps your overall diet.

4. Cook fruits and vegetables as little as possible.

   Heating breaks down fiber; steaming does the least damage to fibers, vitamins, and minerals. Eating foods fresh and in their natural state usually yields the most nutritious results.

5. Keep the skins on apples and potatoes—they add no calories but considerable fiber.

6. Pasta and potatoes and bread—the old taboos in diets—are not fattening and should be brought back into even a weight-losing diet.

   What you have to worry about is what you put on these foods (as long as you eat them in moderation). Pepper, paprika, lemon, or even tomato sauce can add more flavor—and fewer calories— to a baked potato than butter and sour cream. A tomato sauce need not have many calories, especially if you forgo the meat and much of the oil, and instead use garlic and onions and spices to provide the richness and zest.

7. Use fresh fruits instead of cakes and cookies, if you feel a meal is incomplete without dessert.

   Buying luscious fruits all year round is not cheap, but it is an indulgence that is worth far more—and in the long run probably costs less—than purchasing ready-made confections.

8. When you bake your own goodies, use raisins and dates and other fruits as sweeteners rather than sugar.

   Unlike sugar, these fruits also contain other useful nutrients, as well as fiber. They can be added whole, chopped, or ground. Date sugar—a crunchy granule that looks much like brown sugar—can be added to such things as breakfast cereal or yogurt for a touch of sweetness and just a touch of additional fiber.

9. If you can't resist the sweets, try a few of these painless substitutes.

   Frozen yogurt instead of ice cream; plain yogurt instead of sour cream; bittersweet instead of milk chocolate. Not much of a change, but we all have to start somewhere.

10. Bear in mind that sweet foods are high in calories because of their fat as well as sugar content, so they carry all the health hazards of fatty foods. Furthermore, since they contain few nutrients (that's why they're called "empty calories"), sweet foods take up calories in your diet that could be devoted to obtaining the vitamins and minerals that your body needs to keep you alive and ward off disease.

Other Diet Tips for Health

ANTICOLD DIET

The old adage about feeding a cold turns out to be right, if the food you eat is spicy or accompanied with wine.

Spices and hot foods, like chili peppers, garlic, and horseradish, may help clear up colds, asthma, bronchitis, or sinusitis. They irritate the digestive tract, causing a reflex increase in respiratory tract secretions from the nose and lungs. These watery secretions loosen mucus in the airways and flush out potentially troublesome bacteria and viruses. Thus people who eat spicy foods—such as Chinese Hunan or Szechuan as well as Thai, Mexican, Indian, and Pakistani foods—seem to have less chronic obstruction of the lungs than those who don't.

Though evidence is only anecdotal at this point, one doctor at the University of California at Los Angeles who is doing research on this is already advising his bronchitis patients to eat one spicy meal a day and drink plenty of water. For those who can't take the spices, he advises gargling with ten drops of tabasco sauce in a cup of warm water.

Wine, too, contains substances that help fight colds by actually killing cold viruses, according to Canadian virologists. Red wine contains more of these tannins and phenols than white. However, grapes and grape juice contain even more active ingredients than their fermented cousin, and those tannins and phenols can also be found in fruits such as strawberries and raspberries.

STRONG-BONES DIET

Osteoporosis, a condition in which bones become brittle and break easily, comes not only with age (starting after forty-five) but can also be brought on by consuming too little calcium and too much phosphorous.

1. Drink milk and eat milk products.

   If you are worried about the fat content and the calories, choose skim milk and skim milk cheeses, which contain all the nutrients of the whole-milk varieties.

2. Avoid colas and all soft drinks.

   Colas contain phosphorous, which blocks the absorption of calcium. So even if you think you're getting calcium from cheeses, you may not be able to use what you consume if you reach for a soft drink instead of a glass of milk to quench your thirst.

3. Good sources of calcium are skim milk, collard greens, salmon, soybeans and red, black, and white beans as well.

SPORTS DIET

Forget the old high-protein diet many sports trainers used to prescribe. Even muscle-bound weight lifters do not need to load up on meats and proteins.

The best diet for athletes is actually the same high-carbohydrate, low-fat, and low protein diet that is healthiest for all of us.

Carbohydrate loading—the custom of eating large amounts several times a day for three days before a sports event—is useful only for events such as marathons that require a great deal of endurance.

Oddly enough, there is some evidence that drinking a cup of coffee can also aid endurance by causing the release of free fatty acids and sparing some of the glycogen (muscle sugar).

After a race that has involved considerable perspiring, you will have lost salt and zinc. But salt tablets are rarely necessary—before or after—and can make matters worse. You have to secrete about a pint of sweat to lose a gram of salt. Furthermore, after a week of exercising in hot weather, your body begins adjusting to the demands and secretes less salt through sweat than usual.

Normal eating and drinking after a workout should replenish the supply of any lost minerals.

CUT DOWN ON CAFFEINE

Some 5 million Americans drink more than 10 cups of coffee a day. That's too much. Two cups is a safer range.

Coffee has been implicated in heart disease (it seems to increase epinephrine levels in the blood), pancreatic cancer (a Harvard School of Public Health study found a link between coffee but not other forms of caffeine), and increased cigarette smoking (heavy coffee drinkers are three times more likely to smoke than noncoffee drinkers).

To cut down, you first have to know how much caffeine is in the foods—and drugs—you consume.

CAFFEINE CONTENTS

Coffee	100–150 mg per cup
Tea	35–150 mg per cup
Cocoa	50 mg per cup
Cola 12 oz.	50 mg
Midol	Each tablet 32.4 mg (normal dosage is 2 tablets)

CUT ALCOHOL CONSUMPTION

While moderate drinking (less than two ounces a day or twelve cocktails a week) may provide protection against developing heart disease, drinking more than that can cause cirrhosis of the liver, gout, accidents, psychological problems, not to mention the possibility of a variety of cancers. In addition, alcohol can affect male sexual potency and dull the intensity of orgasms for both men and women.

1. Here, as with dietary changes, you must seek help from spouses and friends, committing yourself openly to the idea of cutting down.
2. Start with small goals—cutting back to wine with meals only, for example—and reward yourself when you stick to the goals.
3. Be prepared for the inevitable temptations and work out in advance how you will resist.
4. If the process proves too hard to do alone, seek professional help.
5. Don't watch TV.

Seeing others drink makes it hard to restrain yourself, and alcohol is mentioned in 80 percent of prime-time shows (not to mention commercials). After 9:00 P.M. not one hour goes by without at least three instances of someone using an alcoholic beverage.

Daytime TV has even more alcohol use. The soap operas have an average of six instances per hour of alcohol consumption.

16
Quit Smoking, Start Living

BEFORE WE GET INTO the latest information on what exactly makes smoking so dangerous and how you can go about kicking the habit, it is important to let you in on a new secret: you can quit, and more people do it than the scientific studies up until now have suggested.

Sure, it's hard to quit—smoking, drinking, eating, whatever. And many of us try and fail at first.

But in the end, most people succeed, and succeed largely on their own, with tips from a book or just their own personal systems. Most never make it to formal programs, so their successes in fighting addiction are never registered to balance out the statistics of failure we have come to accept as gospel. That gospel is flat wrong.

In surveying 12,000 people, the Public Health Service found that of the nearly three-quarters of the smokers who had tried to quit, half succeeded.

In a much smaller study by a psychology professor at Columbia University, those who tried to quit on their own were two to three times as successful at quitting as those who sought professional help. And of those who tried to lose weight, over 62 percent were successful in that they currently weighed 10 percent less than when they first tried to lose weight and were now less than 10 percent over their ideal weight.

The new data suggest that quitting proceeds in waves. A large number of people try to stop, and perhaps 10 percent succeed on the first go-around. Then the remainder try again, and perhaps again only 10 percent succeed in quitting for life. By this time, the success rate for the original group is up to 20 percent. On the third day, it's up to 30 percent. And pretty soon, if the originals stick to it, as each quitting effort becomes easier, the vast majority can be destined for success. Remember, trying and trying again does not mean "failure"—it is all part of the normal quitting process.

You can do it all by yourself. But there's no reason for you to have to reinvent the wheel. There are techniques that will make the process easier. Here are some suggestions on how to prepare to quit, how to proceed, how to minimize the discomfort and maximize your chances to reclaim your heart, your lungs, your health.

And for those who aren't quite ready to kick the habit altogether, there are suggestions—and a special diet—that can help you cut down on the number of cigarettes you smoke.

Why Quit—What's All the Furor Over a Little Smoke?

We all know smoking kills. But do you really know . . .
- Nicotine is a poison so lethal that if you were to swallow the amount that can be extracted from five cigarettes, you'd die in three minutes.
- Women who smoke run the same risk of heart attack as men.
- Tobacco use can lead to male impotence. No wonder smokers light up after sex: if they lit up before, there might not be an after.

Smoking is directly responsible for 320,000 deaths a year in the United States. Without it, lung cancer would be a rarity instead of the leading cancer among men and women. Smoking contributes to heart disease, as well as cancers of the lung, esophagus, larynx, pharynx, pancreas, bladder, mouth, and tongue; it leads to chronic bronchitis, emphysema, respiratory infections, and stomach ulcers.

Smoking in pregnancy can retard fetal growth, increase the risk of spontaneous abortion, and impair an infant's normal growth and development.

It seems silly to go on, either with this catalog of ills or with smoking.

What Smoke Does in Your Body

Inhaling any smoke reduces the level of oxygen in the blood, the oxygen that circulates to all the cells in the body to keep them alive. It also stimulates the release of stress chemicals called catecholamines that increase blood pressure, heart rate, and release fatty acids into the blood. The combination of the added hormones and reduced oxygen forces the heart to work much harder than normal. Furthermore, the smoke irritates and damages blood vessels. And the fatty acids that are released eventually form clots in the blood that can block blood to the heart and brain. All these factors increase the chances of heart attacks and strokes.

While tar contains the principal cancer-causing agents in cigarette smoke, it is far from the only dangerous element. It is simply the first to be pinned down as an evil among 2500 compounds that make up smoke, dozens more of which also seem to cause cancer.

Smoke also acts synergistically with other substances—that means when you smoke and take in some other harmful substance, such as alcohol, you run a health risk that is much higher than the sum of the risks. In short, smoke brings out the "best" in other noxious chemicals, giving all of them the multiplied strength to do their worst.

Cigarettes multiply the risks when combined with:

- **The contraceptive pill**—the risk is heart disease and stroke.
- **Alcohol**—the risk is cancer of the larynx, oral cavity, and esophagus.
- **Asbestos**—the risk is lung cancer.
- **Carelessness**—smoking also plays a major role in injuries such as fires and burns; 29 percent of fatal house fires are started by someone who was smoking.

Smokers Make Dangerous Friends

Smokers are not just killing themselves, they're putting their closest friends and relations at risk, too.

Even if you have never lit up yourself, if your spouse or close co-worker smokes around you, after twenty years your respiratory system will suffer all the damages of someone who has smoked eleven cigarettes a day for those twenty years.

And if two smokers live and work together, they are multiplying each other's risks.

A mother (or primary caretaker) who smokes in the house is increasing her child's chances of developing asthma; 18 to 34 percent of asthma cases can be attributed to the mother smoking, according to researchers at Harvard School of Public Health. Children whose parents smoke have twice the incidence of respiratory illness of non-smokers' children. And a Seattle study shows that parents' smoking can lead to children's chronic middle-ear infections as well.

Who's Quitting—What Company Will You Be Keeping?

The smarter you are the more likely you are to quit (or never start). Studies show that the habit is less prevalent among the higher-educated adults. Even among young people, one study by the Institute of Social Research at the University of Michigan found that college-bound seniors were less than half as likely to smoke as those who had no college plans.

Men are quitting—since the 1950s smoking has dropped off from over half of men to around one-third. Women, however, are at it more than ever, from around one-fourth in the 1950s to one-third now. Teenage smoking, after several years of decline, is now on the rise.

There are an estimated 34 million ex-smokers in the United States. A number of surveys have shown that anywhere from 66 to 90 percent of smokers really wish they could kick the habit. So if you're one of the 59 million Americans still puffing away, wishing you could keep your future health from going up in smoke, these tips are for you.

How to Quit

The best technique for quitting—once you have decided to quit—involves cutting down for a short period as you lead up to the day when you will quit completely. This gives you a chance to make the necessary preparations; you're more likely to succeed if you have worked out in advance how to cope with the inevitable temptations and traumas. And at the very least, if you don't stick to your goal to quit completely this time, you will have learned a useful technique for cutting down, you will have given your lungs a break, and you will know how to prepare yourself better so the next attempt may really be your last.

The ten in the ten-day plan that follows is not a magic number. If you feel you need to spend longer cutting down before you take the final step, fine. Or if you decide today that you want to quit, and you don't want to risk losing your resolve, then go ahead and give it your best shot. But for most people, the most important element of a successful quitting scheme is to be able to prepare in advance for those inevitable urges, and know just what to do to overcome them with the least discomfort. This ten-day plan equips you to face the tough times at a controlled pace—not so fast that you panic and feel overwhelmed and not so slow that you lose your willpower.

Ten-Day Quit Smoking Plan: How to Cut Down and Cut It Out

Day 1. The beginning.
1. Decide you want to quit.

No technique will work if you haven't made the basic decision that you really want to quit this time. Make a list of all the good reasons for quitting and all the reasons for continuing to undermine your health by smoking.

If you're still on the fence, afraid to commit yourself, afraid to risk failure, afraid you will get fat if you give up cigarettes, or feel too jittery, bear this in mind:

You have nothing to lose by trying—at the very least you will have given your lungs a temporary break from the irritation and cancerous chemicals in smoke. Lungs are very forgiving—as soon as you remove the smoke they begin repairing damaged cells. So even if you return to smoking, you will have done yourself a little good.

And you have everything to gain if you actually go all the way. In your first year after quitting, you cut your risk for heart attacks by half. Within ten years after quitting, your risks will be back down to those of someone who never smoked. You will be twenty times less likely to suffer cancer than you will if you keep on smoking, and you will come down with fewer pesky little illnesses like colds and the flu. You will not only help yourself live longer but you'll also help those innocent bystanders who live and work around you as well.

As for losing face if you fail, recognize that it takes more guts to try, even if you don't make it right away, than it does to just keep on going as you are.
2. Set a date for when you will quit. Five to ten days should be enough—this plan uses nine days.

Mark the quit day on all calendars you use, at home and in the office.
3. Save all butts of cigarettes you smoke until then and put them in a jar for later.

Day 2. Cut down.

1. Keep a daily diary of every cigarette you smoke, when you smoke it, and what you are doing when you smoke—driving, drinking coffee, drinking alcohol, talking on the phone, after a meal, upon seeing someone else smoke or smelling smoke, and so on.

   Also note for each cigarette, how strong the urge to smoke was on a 1 to 4 scale from weakest to strongest and how much you enjoyed the cigarette, on a 1 to 4 scale from least to most.

   The diary could look something like the one shown below and should be kept tied around your cigarette pack so you can jot down each smoke.

TRACKING THE HABIT

MONDAY

Time of Day	Activity	Urge Rating	Enjoyment Rating
_____	_____	_____	_____
_____	_____	_____	_____
_____	_____	_____	_____
_____	_____	_____	_____

TOTAL SMOKED: _____

2. Enlist the support of your spouse, friends, and co-workers.

   If all your friends and relations smoke, it may be hard to get support from them. Tell them openly that you are going to try to quit and you will need their help when your will weakens. Studies show that openly committing yourself to the goal of quitting as well as getting family support increases the chances for success. (The American Cancer Society has lists of people who will serve as a supportive buddy while you quit.)

Day 3. Continue recording every cigarette you smoke. After two days, you will see patterns of when you smoke and why. Once you understand your habit, you can begin to cut back on those cigarettes you need and enjoy least.

You can also recognize what makes you feel the strongest need to smoke so that you can deliberately imagine yourself doing whatever it is—hearing the phone ring, sitting down to face a pile of paperwork, resting your fork after a pleasant meal—and rehearse substitute behavior that will enable you to resist that urge.

Pick a very specific substitute behavior for each tricky situation: reach for a pencil to fiddle with when the phone rings, drink a glass of water or bubbly seltzer to brace you as you face the pile of paperwork, put a toothpick in your mouth at the end of a meal. Do anything so long as you won't feel as if you are missing something and need to fill the void with smoke.

Day 4. Cut out all the cigarettes that rated a 1 on urge or enjoyment. Count up the number of cigarettes that leaves and parcel out that number for your day's supply. It should be at least a 15 percent cutback.

Day 5. Cut out all the 2-rating cigarettes.

If the rating scale doesn't help you cut down, try setting no-smoking hours during the day—declare that there will be no smoking before 11:00 A.M. or after 10:00 P.M. Then increase the number of no-smoking hours each day. You can also set up no-smoking areas—pronounce the bedroom, or the dining room, or the car off limits. But in all cases, set a limit on the number of cigarettes you will smoke that day and stick to it.

At the very least, resolve not to smoke if you're anywhere near infants or children. You are not only exposing them to dangerous chemicals but setting a bad example as well. Then expand that rule to not smoking in front of any nonsmoker or ex-smoker; if that doesn't help you cut down enough, vow not to smoke in the presence of anyone wearing blue or red. You're in charge; you can set the rules. And who's to say whether it's sillier to light up when the phone rings or put the cigarette out when a red-clad friend walks in?

Day 6. Cut out all the 3-rating cigarettes.

The aim is to get down to as few cigarettes as possible before quitting day—once you get below fifteen cigarettes a day, quitting becomes much easier.

Day 7. Continue the cutdown, using this time to practice your stress-reduction techniques and the various urge-fighting skills you need not only to cut down but to quit. (See tips below and stress-control techniques in chapter 12, "Learning to Love Stress.")

Be prepared to feel uncomfortable as you cut down. Not only are you fighting the nicotine addiction but your body is also beginning to heal itself, and often things get worse before they get better. Soon enough, you will feel better than you ever did while smoking.

Day 8. The day before quitting.
1. This is the day to apply aversion therapy, which seems to help bolster willpower for many.

   The extreme version of aversion. Do not cut down, do not smoke as you used to, smoke until it makes you sick. Double your old level, smoke one right after the other for as long as you can stand it. By the middle of the day you should concentrate intensely on all the unpleasant aspects of smoking: how it hurts your throat, makes your hair and breath stink, saturates your clothes, annoys those around you. Let your imagination go.

If you already have cardiovascular problems, do not try this approach without a doctor's supervision, as rapid smoking can cause great distress.

A milder version of aversion. If you are proceeding well with cutting down, then continue reducing your intake; but as you smoke, you should concentrate on everything unpleasant about it: how the smoke dries your throat, paralyzing cells that wash away infectious bacteria, leaving you vulnerable to sore throats and more serious diseases; how the chemicals in the smoke blacken the lungs, destroy cells in blood vessels, release fats that clog your arteries, and choke off blood to the heart and brain.

Hold the smoke in a little longer as you explore every disgusting aspect of this habit you can possibly conjure.

2. Buy supplies for tomorrow—the substitutes that will help you fight the smoking urge.

Some handy oral substitutes: sugarless gum, a bowl of fruit, fruit juices, a new glass (you can think of it as your "nonsmoker's glass") to hold the fresh water that should be constantly within reach, carrots and celery to munch, tart candy to suck on or chewable vitamin C tablets to crunch on.

Day 9—quitting day. Throw away all cigarettes, remove matches from view. Clean and store ashtrays.

Estimate how much money you will save by the end of the month and the year.

Keep busy—take walks in the fresh air and breathe deeply; even the most polluted air breathed over a year cannot do as much damage as one pack of cigarettes.

Drink plenty of water and juice.

Go to a dentist and have your teeth cleaned—get rid of the old nicotine yellow for good.

Avoid caffeine and alcohol and sweets—they seem to trigger the craving for tobacco.

Brush your teeth after a meal.

Review the benefits of not smoking (refer to the beginning of this chapter if you need reminders).

Go to bed early—it shortens the hours you have to resist smoking and it makes you feel refreshed to face the next day.

Throughout the day, as the urges arise, and at night, if you have any difficulty sleeping, run through the Ten-Second Stress Fix and the other stress-management techniques described in chapter 12.

Treat yourself to something special.

Day 10—the day after—coping with anticlimax and new beginnings. The second day after quitting and many days ahead will involve tougher times than yesterday. The specialness of the Quitting Day is over and now you face the daily trials of keeping your resistance and your spirits up. The struggle begins, but it won't be long. Soon not smoking will become just as much of a habit as smoking used to be.

For now, spend as much time as possible in places where smoking is prohibited: museums, libraries, theaters, churches, department stores. This will help reinforce your resolve.

Mark off on your calendar each day you get through without a cigarette—shade it in with a color or draw a special symbol. The sight of a whole block of these symbols is heartening.

Rehearse exactly what you will say and do when the inevitable occurs: someone offers you a cigarette. Imagine your feelings, your temptations, and your final overcoming of the enticement with the words, "Thanks, but I've just quit," or "Get those out of here, and don't you smoke either—I've just quit and I can't stand the temptation."

And also bear in mind that, while you want at all costs not to let a cigarette touch your lips, if it should happen, it is not the end. One puff does not mean you have to give it all up. You've gone through the hardest part—a slip will make staying off a little harder, but not nearly as hard as throwing up your hands, giving in, and then having to start from Day One again.

Tips on Reducing That Urge to Smoke

These tips are useful for cutting down and for quitting.

1. Change your daily routine.

    You are fighting not only a nicotine addiction but a deeply ingrained set of habits. If you disrupt those habits—eat breakfast in a different chair from the one you usually smoke in, drive to work along a different route that requires more concentration so you won't miss the cigarette—you will find it easier to disrupt the smoking habit as well.

2. Make the cigarettes hard to reach.

   If you're used to reaching for a cigarette before you even get out of bed in the morning, don't leave the pack on the night table.

   At all times, stash the cigarettes somewhere that requires you to move before you smoke. Every delay gives you a second chance to consider whether you really want to smoke or not.

3. Change cigarette brands, and do not buy cartons, only packs.

   Changing not only adds to the disruption of routine, but if you change to a brand you don't like, it will make cutting down and quitting easier.

4. At those times of day and during those activities when you know the urge will be strongest, get up and go out for a walk.

   You don't have to go far—down the hall, up on the elevator to another floor, around the block. Exercise helps distract your yearnings and is also the kind of activity you probably don't associate with smoking.

   If you return to your place and the urge is still strong, go out again. Run, jog, get a drink of water. And tell yourself that when you return, you will concentrate on your work not on cigarettes.

5. Keep a good supply of low-calorie oral substitutes handy: carrots and celery are excellent to munch; so are cucumbers and pickles, sugarless gum, sour lemon drops. For your hands, set up a box of special pencils nearby to keep your hands occupied. Splurge on a colorful set of felt-tip pens that make doodling fun.

6. Use the Ten-Second Stress Fix and other stress-fighting techniques (outlined in chapter 12) throughout the day.

   The urge for a cigarette can increase when you feel under stress. It has been shown that smokers experience a drop in the nicotine levels in their blood under stress which could increase the yearning for a cigarette. Be prepared with an alternative to that urge.

7. Keep a glass of fresh water on your desk or at hand at all times.

   Sometimes those who cut down or stop smoking get a cough. It is a sign that the cilia that line your lungs which were once paralyzed by the smoke during the day are now coming to life and doing their job in cleaning out your lungs. The cough will only last a few weeks, and a drink of water will help the cleaning process. In addition it keeps your hands busy and feels refreshing. (It's an old dieters' trick, as well; so if you're concerned about gaining weight when you quit, keep water handy.)

8. Do not linger after a meal if that's when you are used to lighting up.

Get up and brush your teeth whenever the urge to smoke strikes—the fresh taste this will leave in your mouth will contrast with the stale taste smoking usually leaves and cut the desire. It may seem rude to rise abruptly, but better to be rude for a few weeks than dead prematurely.

9. Talk to yourself positively—encourage yourself when feeling low.

When you feel irritable and nervous and think a cigarette will solve the problem, remind yourself that nobody ever died from nicotine withdrawal—this feeling will pass in a minute.

Repeat encouraging words: "I can do it—I hate smoking and I'm going to stop. I'll be fine as soon as I think of something else." (See chapter 12 for a further discussion of Stress and Stressless Talk.)

10. Avoid alcohol and coffee—these drinks seem to trigger the desire to smoke.

11. Take a whiff of your butt jar—add a bit of water to get the full aromatic effect.

12. Avoid other people who smoke—and turn off the TV.

The power of suggestion in seeing others light up is strong, whether in person or in magazine ads or on TV. Avoidance is safest early on; flip quickly past cigarette ads in magazines. And if you can't resist the tube, at least steer clear of crime and drama shows, where people are more likely to smoke than in situation comedies. Don't expect much sympathy about quitting pangs from your smoking friends. But don't hold off going to those few dedicated friends you selected at the beginning to help you through.

The Smoker's Cut-Down Diet

The major reason people smoke is to get nicotine—that is the chemically addictive element of smoking. And while the urge to smoke can be triggered by circumstances or moods, it strikes primarily when the supply of nicotine in the smoker's blood goes down, usually about half an hour after the last cigarette.

But, if you can keep nicotine in the system longer without increasing the cigarettes smoked, then you may be able to help yourself resist the urge to smoke longer, and thus smoke less.

That's what this diet aims to do.

Researchers at Columbia University and the University of Nebraska College of Medicine have found that the more acidic your diet (and thus the urine you excrete), the faster your body gets rid of nicotine. The more alkaline (or basic) the diet, the longer the nicotine remains. Stress has been shown to increase the acidity of urine, which means that a person under stress is excreting nicotine faster than normal—not hard to see why smokers reach for a cigarette when they're tense. People with a more alkaline blood chemistry smoke less under stress.

Therefore, the more alkaline you make your diet, the easier it should be to cut down on your smoking.

Here are foods to try to supplement your normal diet that will raise your alkalinity and some to avoid, *for a while,* that will raise acidity.

Eat	*Avoid*
Lima beans	Alcohol
Raisins and figs	Dried lentils
Spinach	Chicken and eggs
Almonds	Beef
Carrots	Liver
Celery	Lamb
Grapefruit	Walnuts
Tomatoes	Cheddar cheese
Brewer's yeast	Wheat germ
Vitamin C in the form of sodium ascorbate	Vitamin C in ascorbic acid form

In addition, to reduce the tension and jangled nerves that can accompany withdrawing from cigarettes, make sure you drink plenty of water and eat foods high in the B-complex vitamins. Good sources of the B vitamins are milk, lean meats, poultry, green vegetables, brewer's yeast, wheat germ, whole-grain cereals, and eggs. Although some of these foods are acidic, it is possible, if you compare lists, to get both B vitamins and a more alkaline diet at once.

17
Self-Help Medical Aid

SOMETIMES, no matter how hard you try to prevent accidents and injuries, there's a slipup. Something goes wrong. Here are instructions on how to make them right again—the first steps to take to minimize the damage and the danger and when to seek out a professional.

Life or Death

First things first. To handle life-threatening emergencies, where action has to be taken in the first few minutes or life will be lost, the two things you must know are how to restore breathing and how to get the heart beating.

But as you proceed, remember to listen to the voice inside your head repeating, "Don't panic." It is just as important to the injured person's survival for you to stay outwardly calm and reassuring as it is to know how to administer specific techniques. Reassurance will help the victim respond to treatment and reduce the likelihood of physical and emotional shock, which can be fatal by itself and certainly can complicate any other injury.

Breathing Has Stopped

The first task is to clear the airway.

If the person is unconscious or in the throes of a seizure, it may be that the tongue is obstructing breathing because it has fallen to the back of the throat. Never use your fingers to move the tongue; people have been known to regain consciousness and chomp down hard enough to sever fingers. The following techniques get the tongue to one side, clear the airway, and do not involve risk of being bitten.

HEAD TILT
1. Place your hand under the person's neck.
2. Rest your other hand on his forehead.
3. Now gently lift the neck and push the head back, allowing the mouth to open automatically.

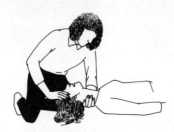

JAW PULL
1. Once the person is on his back, press one hand on his forehead to tilt the head back, and with the other hand grasp the chin to pull the jaw open.

Choking—The Heimlich Maneuver

If the person is eating and suddenly begins gasping for breath, cannot speak, and begins to turn gray-blue, it is quite likely that a piece of food is obstructing the airway. (If it were a heart attack, the person would be able to speak; see chapter 6 for a description of heart attack symptoms, if you are in doubt.) More people die from choking on food than from airplane accidents, snake bites, and electrical shocks put together.

Do not waste time with thumping the person on the back. Debate continues over whether it does any good or whether it can make matters worse. But no one disputes that the Heimlich maneuver is effective. So it is best to begin with Heimlich, and quickly. If the choking victim doesn't get air within four to six minutes, he or she will die.

IF CHOKING PERSON IS STANDING
1. Stand behind the choking person and put your arms around the middle.
2. Make a fist with one hand, thumb side pressing just above his navel and below the rib cage. Clasp your clenched fist with your other hand.
3. Press your fist sharply inward and upward against the person's abdomen. This should compress the air in the lungs and send the trapped food flying out.
4. Repeat if necessary.

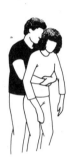

IF THE CHOKING PERSON IS SITTING
1. Stand behind the chair and carry out the maneuver in the same way.
2. If you can't get your arms around the chair and the person, turn the person 90 degrees on the chair (the chair must have no arms) so his back is free of the chair's back, and continue as outlined above.

IF THE CHOKING PERSON IS LYING DOWN
1. Put him on his back.
2. Kneel astride him.
3. Place the heel of one hand above the navel and below the rib cage; put your other hand on top of the first.
4. Press into the abdomen with the same sharp upward thrust used on a standing victim.

IF A CHILD IS CHOKING
1. Try the Heimlich maneuver, only very gently.
2. Or put the child across your knees, or over your arm, head facing down, and thump the back between the shoulder blades more gently than you would with an adult.

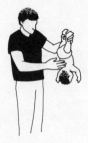
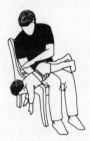

3. You can hold an infant up by the ankles and thump gently on the back.

IF THE CHOKING PERSON IS PREGNANT

Heimlich can still be performed. The area to press is just above the region bulging because of the pregnancy.

MOUTH-TO-MOUTH RESUSCITATION

If the above techniques don't get breathing started again even after the airway has been cleared, then the Kiss of Life is the next step.

1. Place the person flat on his back.
2. Tilt his head back by slipping one hand under the neck and pressing gently with the other on the forehead or by cupping the chin and pressing gently on the forehead as described in the above Head Tilt and Jaw Pull maneuvers.

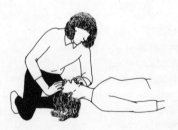

3. Pinch his nostrils closed, using the finger and thumb of the hand still resting on his forehead.
4. Take a deep breath, place your mouth over his, making a tight seal, and exhale quickly four times, hard at first, until you see his chest rise.

5. Rest, to let his chest go down by itself and to see if he resumes breathing.
6. If the person is not yet breathing, continue, giving a breath every 4 or 5 seconds, until he resumes on his own.
7. If the stomach bulges, it may mean air has been pushed into the stomach, too. Turn the person slightly on his side, and be prepared for exhalation of wind or even vomit. Clear the vomit quickly.

FOR CHILDREN AND INFANTS
1. Place your mouth over both their nose and mouth, making a tight seal.
2. Exhale gently, with quick puffs.
3. Give one small breath every 3 seconds.

Drowning Resuscitation

If the person has been dragged out of the water and does not begin breathing, the first step should be mouth-to-mouth resuscitation instantly—it is the most effective of the artificial respiration procedures. If it doesn't get results, you might try administering the Heimlich maneuver to expel water from the lungs, and then try mouth-to-mouth resuscitation again.

If that doesn't work—or in cases where there is injury to the face so you cannot perform mouth-to-mouth—try the following:

1. Turn the person over on his front, place his hands under his head, and turn his head to one side.
2. Kneel at the person's head, spread your hands out on his back just below the shoulder blades.
3. Straighten your arms and rock forward, using your body weight to force the air out of his lungs.
4. Rock back smoothly onto your heels, pulling the person's elbows up past his ears as you rock.
5. Repeat this rocking motion, rhythmically and smoothly—no sudden, jerky movements—about 12 times a minute, until breathing resumes.

CPR—Cardiopulmonary Resuscitation

After a serious accident or a heart attack (see chapter 6 for the symptoms), a person may not only stop breathing but his heart may stop as well. If there is no pulse, the pupils are dilated, and the skin turns blue-gray (skin-color changes will not be discernible in a dark-skinned person), you must apply not only mouth-to-mouth resuscitation but also pressure to restart the heart.

To find out if there is a pulse, put your fingers gently on the windpipe below the chin and then move the fingers slightly to the side of the neck—it is the carotid pulse. If there is none, and no sign of breathing, send someone else for additional help and begin CPR.

1. Place the person on his back, loosen any tight clothing, and kneel to one side of him.
2. Clear airway and carry out mouth-to-mouth resuscitation as outlined above. Start with 2 breaths and then do a chest press.
3. Perform *chest presses:*

     Kneel to the side of the unconscious adult at chest level and locate the sternum or breastbone, the bone running down the center of the chest.

     Place the heel of one hand an inch or two up from the bottom of the sternum, in the center of the chest, stretching fingers up and off the chest wall.

     Place the other hand on top of the first, interlock fingers to help keep from pressing on the chest wall.

     Straighten arms, have your shoulders lined up over the victim's sternum, and press downward 1 or 2 inches.

     Then release pressure completely, but keep hands in place. Repeat.

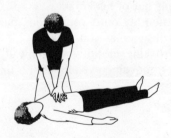

The rhythmic pressure on the lower part of the breastbone presses the heart (which is underneath) against the spine, forcing it to pump blood.

4. The rhythm of the lung inflations and chest presses:

With two rescuers. One should be in charge of the breathing, the other the heart, with both proceeding simultaneously. For each 5 chest compressions there should be 2 lung inflations (carried out on the upstrike of the heart compression). There should be 1 chest press per second.

With one rescuer. If you are alone, alternate 2 lung inflations with 15 heart presses. The heart presses should be faster than 1 per second to get in 80 per minute.

5. Continue until breathing and heartbeat resume.

CPR ON CHILDREN

1. Do not tilt the head *too far back*—infants have more flexible necks and you can block air passages rather than open them.
2. Use shallower more frequent breaths than with an adult—1 every 3 seconds—covering the mouth and nose with your mouth.
3. For the chest press, use only the heel of 1 hand or, with infants, 2 fingers. Press less deeply—from ½ inch to 1½ inches depending on the victim's age. Press at a faster rate—100 to 120 presses per minute.
4. The rhythm remains the same, 2 breaths after every fifth chest press.

While you may be able to carry out CPR on the basis of this description, it is best to be trained first by someone experienced. If you know someone you live with is at risk for a heart attack, don't delay in getting the training before an emergency.

Recovery Position for the Unconscious

If you have done all you can for the victim, and he is breathing but still has not regained consciousness, place in the following position to ease breathing and to prevent fluids like saliva or vomit from collecting in the throat.

Do not use this position if you suspect spine injury.

1. Loosen any tight clothing.

2. Cup the victim's face with your hand to protect the head as you pull his hip up and over, so he is halfway between being on his front and his side. Turn the head to the side.
3. Bend his top knee and arm to keep him from rolling onto his face.

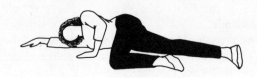

Bleeding—Cuts, Wounds

1. For nearly all bleeding wounds, no matter how severe, the most effective measure to stop the blood flow is to push the edges of the wound together and apply pressure to the wound until the blood clots. (Tourniquets are rarely necessary unless an entire limb is severed.)
2. Get the bleeding person to lie down and position the bleeding limb or body part so that it is higher than the head, then the brain will not lose its blood supply.
3. Once the blood flow eases, apply a bandage (a scarf or handkerchief will do until you can get professional help) to maintain firm pressure but do not make it tight enough to cut off circulation.
4. Once the bleeding has stopped, clean the wound and apply ice to reduce swelling.
5. When do you need a stitch or a visit to the doctor?

Most cuts less than an inch long do not require stitches or a doctor. But if the bleeding continues to soak through a dressing, or if the injured person develops a fever, swollen lymph glands, numbness, increased pain, or red streaks around the wound, you should contact a doctor immediately.

BROKEN BONES OR FRACTURES

Is it broken?

You can't always tell without an X ray. If the person cannot move or put his or her weight on an injured part, or if it is misshapen or very painful, treat it as if it were broken or fractured.

1. Do not force a dislocation back, unless you have been specifically trained to do so.
2. Try to immobilize that part with a splint so you can move the person safely to get professional help. Folded newspapers, magazines, cloth-covered slats of wood can be used as impromptu splints. Ties, scarves, or belts can hold the splint in place.
3. Treat any bleeding (as described above).
4. Keep the person warm, watch for signs of shock, and do not offer any food or drink in case the broken bone will need to be reset under an anesthetic.
5. If there is severe pain in the neck or back, tingling and loss of sensation in the limbs, there may be spinal injury. Do not move the person unless you can slip him onto a rigid surface (a table, a removed door) and keep the body straight.

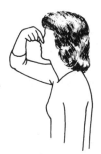

NOSEBLEEDS

Simply squeeze the soft part of the nose between thumb and finger for 15 to 20 minutes without interruption. Once bleeding stops, do not blow the nose, as you may dislodge the clot.

Burns

1. Remove the source of heat—put out flames or, in the case of a scalding or a chemical burn, remove soaked or still-hot clothing. If a person's clothing is on fire, get him to the ground to keep the flames from rising to the head, but do not roll him over and over again— smother the flames with a coat or a rug or a blanket. If burning or smoldering clothing can be removed, it should be ripped off, as it is continuing to burn the tissue. But if the clothing is sticking to the skin, or has cooled after a fire burn, leave it on; the fire has sterilized it and it will protect the burned area.

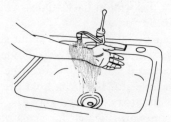

2. Cool the skin—run burned area under cold water for 10 minutes to an hour.
3. Remove all jewelry or anything constricting before the area begins to swell.
4. Do not apply fluffy cotton, tissues, or any ointment, oil, butter, or powder to the burns.
5. If it is a small burn, you can wash the surrounding area with mild soap and water and apply a sterile, medicated burn ointment and wrap it loosely with sterile gauze so it will not become infected but can still breathe.
6. If it is a severe burn, covering a large area, do not try to clean it with anything but water; and do not burst any blisters that form.
7. Wrap a badly burned individual loosely in a clean sheet, moisten lips and give small sips of water to combat fluid loss, and get him to a hospital immediately. Be prepared for him to go into shock.

Shock

Someone who has been burned or cut and has lost a great deal of blood is likely to go into shock. So might a person who has undergone extreme pain, an electrical shock, a heart attack, a burst appendix, extreme allergic reaction, or emotional trauma—all of which can interfere with the supply of blood to crucial organs. Shock itself can be fatal, so it is necessary to recognize the early signs and treat it quickly.

Shock's symptoms:

- Faintness or feeling of giddiness
- Rapid, shallow breathing
- Thirst
- Pale, clammy skin
- Excessive sweating
- Fast but weak pulse
- Blurring of vision

What to do:

1. Handle the underlying cause of the shock—burn, injury, heart attack.
2. Have the person lie down and raise his feet above the level of his head to improve the blood supply to the brain.
3. Moisten his lips with water or give small sips of water.
4. Give mouth-to-mouth resuscitation if this proves necessary.
5. Keep him warm, but not too warm, as you get him to professional help.

Fainting

Conditions that produce shock may also cause fainting.

1. Get the person about to faint to sit down. Loosen tight clothes and gently lean head down toward the knees to get blood to the brain.
2. Tell the person to relax, breathe deeply, and flex leg muscles to get blood circulating. You can also massage arms, wrists, legs (movements should be in the direction of the heart) to stimulate blood circulation manually.
3. If the person faints, get him into the shade, and put him in the Recovery Position.
4. Recovery should be swift. You should be soothing, as the disturbing event or pain that triggered the incident in the first place may still be vivid.

Electrical Shock

An electrical current may leave only a small external mark, but it can do a great deal of internal damage. It can stop breathing, stop the heart, and extensively damage tissue deep inside.

1. Get the victim away from the electrical source—*but not with your bare hands.* The electricity will travel right through you as well. (This does not apply to a lightning victim; only someone still attached to the source of power.)

   Use a dry material that does not conduct electricity, such as wood or paper or rubber—a stick, a broom, a plunger, a rolled-up newspaper, a piece of furniture like a chair or small table.

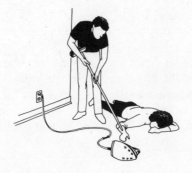

2. If you can't move the person, shut off the electrical power.
3. If the person is not breathing, start mouth-to-mouth resuscitation.
4. If there is no heartbeat, begin CPR.
5. If the person is breathing but unconscious, put him in the Recovery Position and get medical assistance.

Bites and Stings

Insect and animal bites can range from annoying to fatal. Here is the action to take with the most common varieties.

ANIMAL BITES

1. Human bites are as dangerous as animal bites (risking tetanus and other infections); both should be cleaned off (use tincture of iodine).
2. See a doctor—if you haven't had a tetanus booster recently, you'll need an antitetanus shot.
3. If possible, catch the animal and have it tested for rabies.

INSECT BITES OR STINGS

Spiders. Few are poisonous and even those are most dangerous primarily to children, the elderly, and the ill.

If you have extreme pain after a spider bite, apply a cold compress and see a doctor.

Bees, wasps, and hornets, and other insects. Remove the stinger (only the honeybee leaves one) by scraping with a fingernail or knife—tweezers force additional venom into the wound.

Wash the area with soap and water, apply a cold compress, and rest so as not to spread the insect venom. A paste of bicarbonate of soda or meat tenderizer and water, applied to the skin, can help ease the pain.

If the sting is in the mouth, rinse mouth with a solution of one teaspoon of bicarbonate of soda in a tall glass of water. Apply ice.

Jellyfish stings. These can cause a painful burning sensation and swelling but are rarely dangerous. Apply cold compresses for the pain and swelling and calamine lotion later for itching.

Allergic reactions. Symptoms for an allergic reaction to a sting— which usually occur within 20 minutes—are severe swelling of the eyes, lips, tongue, and other parts of the body far from the sting; dry cough followed by a tightening in the throat or chest; nausea, vomiting; dizziness, difficulty breathing; hives on the body; shock; and unconsciousness.

Make the stung person comfortable and get medical help quickly.

SNAKEBITES

Nonpoisonous. Most snakes are not poisonous. Their bites reveal four rows of teeth in the upper jaw and two rows in the lower jaw. If severe pain does not occur immediately followed by serious swelling and discoloration of the skin, then:

- Keep the victim from moving more than necessary.
- Position the bitten area below the heart.
- Clean the wound as you would for an animal bite.
- Get to a doctor.

Poisonous. The most common poisonous snakes in North America are copperheads, moccasins, rattlesnakes, cottonmouths, and coral snakes. Get to know what each looks like.

A bite will cause severe pain, swelling, shortness of breath, discoloration of the skin, possibly nausea or vomiting and shock.

- Remove all jewelry, as the limbs may swell.
- Place tight bands (using a scarf or a belt) above and below the bite to inhibit circulation of the venom, but do not block circulation completely. Remove the bands for a couple of minutes every 15 minutes.
- Make a single cut (not an *X*) over each fang mark parallel to the length of the arm or leg, not across. (Use a knife or razor blade sterilized in a flame.) Suck out the venom and spit it out. Do not do this if you have sores in the mouth; merely squeeze the venom out.

- Keep the victim still and calm to slow the circulation of the poison. Do not give aspirin or anything to eat or drink. Treat for shock, if necessary.
- Capture the snake or get a good look at it, if possible. The identity of the snake affects the treatment; there are antivenom serums.
- Get to an emergency room.

Poisonings

1. Grab the item you believe the person swallowed and call your state poison control center with the bottle or box or ingredient label in hand. Or at least know the brand name of the substance.
2. Treatment varies according to the nature of the poison.

   Corrosives. For substances that are acidic or alkaline or petroleum-based (dishwasher detergent, lye, drain and oven cleaners, cleaning fluid, insect spray), administering water helps dilute the effects. Rinse the mouth with water and have the child drink water. Do not pour water into an unconscious person—you may choke him. Do not give milk, egg, or oily substances to drink, no matter what the manufacturer's antidote instruction may say.

   Do not induce vomiting—this may aggravate the damage.

   Noncorrosive poisons. If the poison center advises, you should induce vomiting with fingers down the throat or syrup of ipecac. Avoid using salt water as this can be dangerous in itself. (Medicines, poisonous plants, cigarettes are examples of noncorrosive poisons.)
3. If the person is unconscious, take him to the hospital and take along for analysis any samples of the substance ingested.

Seizures

Epilepsy or drug overdose as well as drug or alcohol withdrawal can induce seizures.

1. Keep the victim from falling, but don't try to restrain the jerky movements and rigidity that occur.
2. Put something between the teeth—a comb, a small roll of paper, a stick—to keep victim from biting the tongue and to keep

the tongue from falling back and obstructing the airway. Do not use your hand; you could be bitten.

3. Loosen clothing to make sure breathing is kept easy.
4. Let the victim rest comfortably afterward. Seizures leave victims exhausted.
5. Get help.

Sprains, Strains, Sports Injuries

If it is at all possible that a sprain is actually a broken or fractured bone, treat it as such.

If you know you've simply pulled, pushed, or strained beyond your limits (or in the interval between the injury and when you can get to a doctor), the best advice is RICE:

R   Rest.
I   Ice relieves pain and reduces swelling and bleeding.
C   Cold compress of ice should be wrapped in a bandage so it can stay in place for 20 to 30 minutes; then it should be removed for 15 minutes; then reapplied for the next 30 minutes. Continue applying and removing the compress for 3 hours.
E   Elevation of the injured part above the level of the heart allows gravity to drain the excess fluid from the injured area.

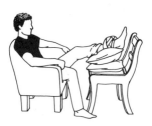

Continue elevating the injured part and applying cold compresses periodically for the next 24 hours. If pain and swelling persist for 2 days after the injury, then apply heat.

If the pain is too severe to move the injured part or if it persists for a couple of weeks or doesn't heal in 3 weeks, call a doctor.

After the initial full day of ice treatment, you can begin soaking the strained area in hot water for 15 minutes twice a day. You can also massage the area to speed recovery.

Index